· · *Praise for* · ·

DODGING THE **TOXIC BULLET**

"An excellent overview for everyone who must
know more about the future of health and the planet."

DR. RICHARD J. JACKSON, MD, UCLA School of Public Health

"A well-written, well-researched guide on how to protect oneself
and one's family from a range of environmental health hazards."

DR. ERIC CHIVIAN, MD, Director, Center for Health and the Global Environment, Harvard Medical School

"Amidst the complex stew of facts, beliefs, and rumors about
human health and the environment comes David Boyd's
clear guidance regarding environmental causes of disease.
It is a fascinating, dramatic, and necessary book."

DR. KARL-HENRIK ROBÈRT, MD, oncologist and founder of The Natural Step

"Boyd brilliantly exposes the womb-to-tomb risks in
everything from bad air to bad diets but . . . gives us the
practical steps to save our planet and ourselves!"

TERRY TAMMINEN, author of *Lives per Gallon: The True Cost of Our Oil Addiction*

"For pregnant and breastfeeding women or
any parent of young children, this is an essential resource."

DR. ELIN RAYMOND, MD, Department of Obstetrics and Gynaecology, University of Toronto

"A wonderful guide to making our food, air, and water safer.
Boyd offers excellent advice while showing us something more
important still: how to become advocates for planetary survival."

GIDEON FORMAN, Canadian Association of Physicians for the Environment

"A highly sensible guide with easy, available tips and ideas.
I can't wait to institute these ideas in my household!"

DR. KEVIN CHAN, MD, Faculty of Medicine, University of Toronto

"A delightfully practical guide on how individuals in a polluted world can take charge of their health."

"Boyd provides plenty of practical pointers that succeed in passionately promoting hope in our ability to protect ourselves, our families, and our planet."

"Essential reading for any parent or concerned citizen. Boyd's writing is accessible, intelligent, informative, and balanced."

"This is precisely the sort of book people need to deal with our increasingly toxic society."

"Knowledge is power, and this book is packed! It is an empowering book for healthier people, happier households, and a healthier world."

"A beautifully written yet practical guide that everyone should read. Packed with wisdom and knowledge, if we all followed these recommendations our health and the health of our planet would improve remarkably."

"As a medical doctor involved in caring for people suffering from various health conditions related to adverse environmental exposures, I am grateful for this important work."

DODGING
THE TOXIC
BULLET

HOW TO PROTECT
YOURSELF FROM EVERYDAY
ENVIRONMENTAL HEALTH HAZARDS

DAVID R. BOYD

Foreword by DAVID SUZUKI

 David Suzuki Foundation

 GREYSTONE BOOKS
D&M PUBLISHERS INC.
Vancouver/Toronto/Berkeley

Greystone Books
An imprint of D&M Publishers Inc.
2323 Quebec Street, Suite 201
Vancouver BC Canada V5T 4S7
www.greystonebooks.com

The David Suzuki Foundation
219−2211 West 4th Avenue
Vancouver, BC Canada V6K 4S2

Library and Archives Canada Cataloguing in Publication
Boyd, David R. (David Richard), 1964−
Dodging the toxic bullet: how to protect yourself from everyday
environmental health hazards / David R. Boyd.

Co-published by the David Suzuki Foundation.

Includes bibliographical references and index.
ISBN 978-1-55365-454-4

1. Environmental toxicology—Popular works.   2. Environmental health—Popular works.
I. David Suzuki Foundation   II. Title.
RA565.B69 2010   615.9′02   C2009-906137-6

Editing by Barbara Tomlin
Text design by Naomi MacDougall
Printed and bound in Canada by Friesens
Printed on acid-free paper that is forest friendly
(100% post-consumer recycled paper) and has been processed chlorine free
Distributed in the U.S. by Publishers Group West

We gratefully acknowledge the financial support of the Canada Council for the Arts,
the British Columbia Arts Council, the Province of British Columbia through the Book
Publishing Tax Credit, and the Government of Canada through the Book Publishing
Industry Development Program (BPIDP) for our publishing activities.

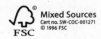

Mixed Sources
Cert no. SW-COC-001271
© 1996 FSC
FSC

This book is dedicated to my daughter, Meredith,
my niece, Sonje, my nephew, Seamus,
and all of the world's children.
It's also dedicated to the memory of Sam.
Healthy kids need a healthy planet.

CONTENTS

PREFACE

LIKE ALMOST EVERYONE, I've experienced the pain of losing loved ones to unexpected illnesses. My mother, an amazing woman who single-handedly raised two boys, was killed by breast cancer when she was barely sixty. Cancer killed my Uncle Bill and my Aunt Anne, a pair of kind and hardworking farmers, well before their lives should have ended. My cousin Mary gave birth to Sam, a boy who suffered from lissencephaly, a rare affliction in which the brain lacks its regular deep folds. Sam lived only two years, but made a profound and lasting impression on our entire family. The daughter of friends suffered from a brain tumor discovered before her tenth birthday. Another friend was diagnosed with breast cancer before she turned forty. These could be random events, attributable to genetic variability and plain bad luck. Or they could be part of the invisible epidemic—the onslaught of disease and illnesses caused by the environmental hazards that are everywhere in today's world, though we can rarely see or sense them.

The invisible epidemic, and the shadows it has cast, haunt me. During nearly twenty years of practising and teaching environmental law, I focused much of my energy and attention on the health of ecosystems rather than people. The connections between the environment and human health were too personal, too painful to contemplate. Then, two events opened the door for me. The first was the birth of my daughter,

Meredith. As every parent can attest, the arrival of a newborn provokes not only joy but unprecedented neuroses about all kinds of potential threats, including environmental risks. The second was the opportunity to fulfill a lifelong dream—pursuing a doctoral degree. I was able to study with experts in toxicology, epidemiology, and environmental health at the University of British Columbia. It was stunning to learn how little we really know about environment-health connections and how grossly inadequate our system of laws and policies is at protecting our health—and our children's health—from environmental hazards. I began my studies believing that in the twenty-first century, following our disastrous experiences with tobacco, asbestos, lead, and other toxic substances, we surely must have learned from the lessons of the past. Unfortunately, I was wrong.

Motivated to protect my daughter and armed with new knowledge, I published seven reports on health and environmental issues with the David Suzuki Foundation, including comparisons of air, water, and food safety standards in Canada, the U.S., Australia, and Europe, studies of pesticide poisonings and radon, an under-rated threat to indoor air quality, and a blueprint for a national environmental health strategy for Canada. These reports hit a nerve. Organizations ranging from the Canadian Cancer Society and the Canadian Public Health Association to the Conference Board of Canada weighed in on the need for stronger government action to protect our health and the environment. The media displayed a voracious appetite for stories linking ecological degradation and people's health. Along the way, almost every person I spoke with about health and the environment asked me the same question: *What can I do?*

This book represents my best effort to answer this question. The good news is that there are many simple steps we can take to protect our health from everyday environmental hazards. But this book is also about going beyond self-interest. This book is about protecting the health and well-being of people without the means to protect themselves, including children, the poor and socially marginalized, and future generations.

The need to take a broader, more inclusive approach was driven home for me several years ago, while visiting family in Ontario. Along with my wife, Margot, who is also an environmental lawyer, I was invited to go on a Toxic Tour of Sarnia, Canada's so-called Chemical Valley. Our host was a courageous community activist named Ron Plain who was working with a group called Environmental Defence. Ron is also a member of the Aamjiwnaang First Nation, whose reserve is located on the outskirts of Sarnia. His ancestors have lived in this area for at least six thousand years.

It was beyond shocking to drive around Sarnia for several hours, stopping at one massive chemical complex after another. There were hundreds of smokestacks belching pollutants into the air. More than sixty major petrochemical and chemical plants are located within a 25-kilometer (15-mile) radius of the community, pumping out hundreds of thousands of tonnes of toxic chemicals annually. We parked briefly outside a vinyl chloride plant where we all felt like gagging, the chemical stench was so powerful. We walked beside a small creek where a sign warned "Keep Out. Talfourd Creek contains toxic substances known to cause serious health risks." We stopped for lunch at the Leaky Tank Truckstop, where I was unable to eat my grilled cheese sandwich and fries because my stomach was tied in knots. We marveled at the twisted sense of humor behind the name of the restaurant and the wall-sized mural of an eighteen-wheeler leaking fluorescent toxic chemicals onto the highway. We stared in disbelief at the former location of the Aamjiwnaang daycare center, right across the highway from several chemical factories. We ended the tour by walking quietly around an Aboriginal cemetery fenced in on three sides by petrochemical plants.

My body rebelled. I've always been blessed with good, even robust physical health, allowing me to complete marathons, ultramarathons, and Ironman triathlons. In my whole life, I've only had two or three headaches, and one of those was due to an ill-advised decision to fast for thirty hours to raise money for an African relief project (a good cause, but not a task suited to my hyperactive metabolism). But after just a couple of hours on the Toxic Tour, my eyes felt as though they'd been rubbed with sandpaper. My throat was raw and my head throbbed with a debilitating headache. In time those symptoms eased, but to this day my heart is sickened by what I saw. In one of the wealthiest, best educated, most technologically advanced nations in the world, with an international reputation for being socially progressive, was one of the most disgraceful displays of human indifference that I have ever seen. If a couple of hours in the poisoned atmosphere of Chemical Valley was enough to make me feel ill, what kind of health problems must be endured by the people who live there?

Our comfortable lifestyle carries a prodigious cost, paid by people who live in places like Sarnia. My Toxic Tour experience illustrates why it's not enough to take actions to protect ourselves and our families from environmental hazards. We also have a moral obligation to ensure that governments and industries take the necessary steps to ensure that everyone is adequately protected from health threats. Places like Chemical Valley violate people's fundamental right to live in a healthy environment. They are a stain on our collective conscience that needs to be scrubbed clean with stronger laws to protect present and future generations and with fair compensation to those who have shouldered a disproportionate burden of society's pollution. Deaths and illnesses caused by exposure to environmental hazards are preventable, not inevitable.

ACKNOWLEDGMENTS

I COULD NOT HAVE written this book without the support of an amazing network of friends and colleagues. Thanks to Dr. David Bates, Dr. Ray Copes, Dr. Hadi Dowlatabadi, and Dr. Milind Kandlikar for teaching me about the finer points of environmental health. Thanks to Dr. Amir Attaran, Dr. Jeanette Boyd, Dr. Kevin Chan, Dr. Stephen Genuis, Lisa Gue, Dr. Scott Harrison, Dr. Richard Jackson, Dr. Faisal Moola, Dr. Peter Paré, Dr. Daniel Rainham, Ann Rowan, Dr. Terre Satterfield, Dr. Meg Sears, Dr. Colin Soskolne, Barry Truax, and Dr. Scott Wallace for their helpful guidance, feedback, and support along the way. More gratitude than mere words can convey is due to Margot and Meredith who made sure that research and writing were balanced with healthy doses of family, play, and beach time.

FOREWORD

IN HER SEMINAL work *Silent Spring*, published in 1962, Rachel Carson documented the unexpected consequences of the widespread use of pesticides, especially DDT, which becomes more concentrated as it moves up the food chain and which ultimately pushed several species of eagles, falcons, and hawks to the brink of extinction. Despite this discovery, we continue to pour toxic substances into our air, water, and soil.

Yet air, water, and the land are part of a single system in nature. Virtually every chemical discharged into the atmosphere anywhere on Earth can be detected at the South Pole, and lake trout in the alpine lakes at Banff National Park in Canada—to name one example—are loaded with toxic pesticides used in Russia. Meanwhile, rates of asthma, breast cancer, prostate cancer, and other illnesses linked to environmental degradation continue their catastrophic rise.

We breathe and then filter air every minute of our lives. Without air, we are dead in a couple of minutes, yet we pour vast quantities of toxins into the air all over the planet. We must consume water daily, yet we dump toxic substances into water to be diluted away. We get every bit of our nutrition from plants and animals, yet we spray pesticides onto the soil, dump chemical wastes into the earth, and even spray or inject highly toxic chemicals into the very plants and animals we will ingest.

Through aboriginal people, I have learned that there is no environment "out there," separate from us. We *are* air, water, and earth, because they are in us and circulating through us. Whatever we do to these sacred elements, we do to ourselves. Our health and well-being mirror the state of the biosphere.

In addition, every year thousands of new chemicals are introduced, most of which have never been adequately tested for how they might affect living organisms. Many of these chemicals are contained in items we use in our homes, including cleaning agents, paints, and cosmetics.

After watching a documentary program on the terrible biological effects of compounds leaching from some kinds of plastics, I said to my wife, "We have to get rid of plastic from our home." Well, dream on, Suzuki. Plastics are contained in everything from baby bottles to toys to water containers, clothing, and all manner of products. Each of us carries several pounds of plastic and dozens of toxic substances dissolved in our bodies. Through our pervasive pollution of the planet, we have inadvertently polluted ourselves, with deadly consequences for our health.

This book contains vital information about how to minimize our exposure to harmful products and find safe replacements for them. It is a desperately needed guide that will help us protect ourselves, but we must also realize that as a society we cannot continue to unload our toxic debris into our air, water, and soil and to manufacture products out of toxic substances. As David Boyd makes clear, when we learn to treat the planet and all of its sacred elements with reverence and respect, the Earth will be healthier and so will we.

David Suzuki

1 ENVIRONMENTAL HEALTH 101

Our behavior is the result of a basic failure to recognize that human beings are an inseparable part of Nature and that we cannot damage it severely without severely damaging ourselves.

Eric Chivian, MD, and Aaron Bernstein, MD,
editors of *Sustaining Life: How Human Health Depends on Biodiversity*

LOOK AT YOUR hands, your face, your body. Think about your heart, your lungs, your brain. Contemplate the development of an infant from the ecstatic moment of conception—when a sperm fertilizes an egg—to the first labored breath at birth. Human beings are extraordinary animals, marvelously complex, even verging on miraculous. Scientists estimate that there are 100 *trillion* cells in the average adult human body, somehow working in synchrony so that we can breathe, think, feel, and love.

With just one exception, every atom, molecule, and element that makes up your body was once part of a star, pulsating away somewhere in the universe billions of years ago. When stars exploded in supernovas, they burst into enormous clouds of dust and gases that eventually came together to form the Earth, and much later, our bodies. All of the basic building blocks of human life—the iron in your blood, the oxygen in your muscles, the calcium in your bones and teeth—are recycled materials from stars. The sole exception is hydrogen, which was generated by the big bang, roughly 14 billion years ago. Thus the hydrogen atoms in your body are as old as the universe itself. The notion that we are stardust may sound fanciful but it is factual. It is physics, not metaphysics.

While we may, technically speaking, be made from recycled stardust, we are constantly replenishing ourselves through the air we breathe, the water we drink, the food we eat, and to a lesser extent, the stuff we touch. It is for this reason that citizens of the twenty-first century are haunted by concerns about the pervasive pollution and toxic contamination of the planet. Pollution is everywhere, not just in city centers and industrial areas. Toxic chemicals can be found at both the South and the North Pole, in remote national parks, on the peaks of mountains, and in the dark abyssal depths of the oceans. Human ingenuity run amok has created thousands of compounds that Nature previously never experienced. Twenty-first century environmental contaminants are often, though not always, undetectable to the human senses. We may be unable to see the pollution in the air, taste the pathogens and chemicals in the water, or smell the pesticides in the food. Our sensory organs have not evolved rapidly enough to protect us from the dangers we have engineered. But we understand, instinctively, that these substances are entering our bodies and may be causing harm.

Human ingenuity run amok has created thousands of compounds that Nature previously never experienced

At our peril, we have ignored warnings from pre-eminent scientists that our destiny is inextricably intertwined with the well-being of the Earth. We treat air, water, and soil as though the planet has an infinite capacity to absorb our waste and pollution. We consume natural resources as though there are no limits, and bury our heads in the sand about the eventual consequences of our actions. Our assumptions, our economics, and our self-ordained dominion over the Earth are woefully misguided. The toxic substances we dump into the environment inevitably boomerang back to us through the air we breathe, the water we drink, the food we eat, and the things we make. We are part of, not separate from, Nature.

If a doctor took a blood sample from every member of your family and sent it to a laboratory, it is almost certain, based on studies from the U.S., Canada, Australia, and Europe, that testing would identify a witches' brew of contaminants: pesticides, flame retardants, stain repellants, rocket fuel residues, heavy metals, and other chemicals. This toxic cocktail, known as your body burden, could even include extremely hazardous substances banned years ago by industrialized nations, such as dioxins and polychlorinated biphenyls (PCBs).

In the U.S., 100% of individuals test positive for perchlorate residues, a toxic additive used in rocket fuel. Bisphenol A or BPA, used in myriad plastic products today, turns up in 93% of Americans, with higher concentrations in children and women. Perfluorinated chemicals (PFCs), used in stain repellants for countless consumer products, are found in 98% of Americans. Although it is hard to believe and heart-breaking to contemplate, even newborn babies are contaminated. In one study, an average of 287 different industrial contaminants were detected in blood taken from the umbilical cords of American infants. Recent studies reveal that babies with higher levels of the pesticide hexachlorobenzene in their bodies at birth (due to maternal exposure) face a higher risk of obesity before the age of six.

Can contaminants measured in parts per million or even parts per billion be harmful to your health? Industry clings to the claim that such small concentrations of chemicals cannot possibly be harmful. They are wrong. Although the mere presence of a toxic substance in your body does not necessarily mean that you will become ill, exposure to some substances at tiny concentrations can produce adverse health effects. For certain toxic substances—some carcinogens such as dioxins and benzene, and many endocrine-disrupting chemicals—there is no completely safe amount of exposure. The pesticide atrazine, which is found in American, Canadian, and Australian drinking water supplies, causes sexual organ deformities and reproductive problems in frogs at concentrations measured in just a few parts per billion. Scientists do not yet know whether exposure to atrazine at similar concentrations affects human health. However, the European Union prohibits all uses of atrazine because of concerns about health and environmental effects, whereas atrazine continues to be one of the most heavily used pesticides in the U.S., Canada, and Australia.

The hazardous substances found in air, food, soil, water, and consumer products are linked to premature death and a lengthy list of adverse health effects including cancer, cardiovascular disease, asthma, chronic obstructive pulmonary disease, developmental disorders, gastrointestinal illnesses, neurodegenerative diseases such as Alzheimer's and Parkinson's, permanent decreases in IQ, premature birth, birth defects, immune system suppression, and reproductive problems. Of growing concern are endocrine-disrupting chemicals (also known as hormone disruptors and gender benders). These substances mimic naturally occurring hormones, leading to reproductive problems (e.g., reduced fertility, reproductive tract abnormalities, skewed male/female sex ratios, miscarriage), early puberty, brain and behavior disorders, impaired immune functions, and cancer.

According to the World Health Organization (WHO), between 25% and 33% of deaths and illnesses in the world today are linked to environmental factors. The proportion is higher in developing nations because of problems such as infectious diseases caused by unsafe drinking water and lack of access to basic sanitation. Nevertheless, in 2007 WHO estimated that 398,000 deaths in the U.S., 36,000 deaths in Canada, and 22,000 deaths in Australia could be attributed to environmental hazards annually. In these three nations, the overall proportion of disease attributed to environmental factors ranges from 13% to 16%. Because of knowledge gaps and limits to WHO's study, these are probably underestimates.

In some cases, the connections between environmental factors and adverse health outcomes are direct and uncontroversial. For example, exposure to asbestos is undeniably a cause of lung cancer, mesothelioma (a deadly form of cancer), and asbestosis (a degenerative lung disease). Air pollution is clearly connected to heart and lung disease. Similarly, there is incontrovertible proof that when young children are exposed to lead they face elevated risks of neurological damage that can last a lifetime. In other cases, the environment-health connections continue to be the subject of intensive research and debate, such as contentious evidence linking pesticide exposures to breast cancer or conflicting studies about the relationship between cell phone use and brain cancer.

It is understandable that there is uncertainty about the exact nature of some links between exposure to environmental hazards and the onset of disease. As Albert Einstein observed, "We still do not know one-thousandth of one percent of what Nature has revealed to us." When it comes to human health, many different factors—lifestyle, diet, genetics, quality of medical care, and socio-economic status, to name just a few—interact over long periods of time. Uncertainty also stems from the fact that comprehensive health studies have never been conducted for the majority of chemicals used today. Another reason for the uncertainty relates to a disturbing Catch-22. For obvious ethical reasons scientists cannot carry out experiments on humans in order to learn about the adverse health effects associated with exposure to toxic substances. And yet we are all being exposed to thousands of chemicals in what amounts to a massive scientific experiment. As diseases and deaths occur, toxicologists and epidemiologists struggle to piece together what is happening. It is a daunting task that continues to yield unpleasant surprises, as the connection between pollution, obesity, and diabetes demonstrates (see page 14).

Air pollution is clearly connected to heart and lung disease

POLLUTION, OBESITY, AND DIABETES ‹‹

SCIENTISTS ARE DISCOVERING connections between pollution, obesity, and diabetes. These connections are profoundly important because for the first time in the modern era, today's children may experience shorter lives and poorer health than their parents. The main culprit behind this shocking development is diabetes, which in turn is linked to obesity. Rates of obesity are skyrocketing. One in three children born today will be afflicted by diabetes unless current trends are reversed. The risk is even higher for some groups, including Aboriginal people, Hispanic Americans, and African Americans. Being diagnosed with diabetes before your fortieth birthday can reduce your life expectancy by ten to fifteen years.

Three scientific breakthroughs demonstrate environmental connections to obesity and diabetes. First, scientists studying the adverse effects of a toxic substance called tributyltin (TBT) on frogs' reproductive systems were surprised when the frogs became extremely obese. The scientists realized that TBT affects the hormone systems of animals in ways that trigger accelerated fat production. Studies have confirmed that several endocrine-disrupting chemicals contribute to fat production. Second, researchers discovered that people with high levels of persistent organic pollutants in their bodies are up to thirty-eight times more likely to suffer from diabetes than people with low body burdens of these pollutants. Third, scientists learned that exposure to some pollutants can cause changes in the way an individual's genes function, and that these changes are passed on, causing obesity in future generations. These discoveries illuminate new environment-health connections and support calls for stronger government intervention to protect people from endocrine-disrupting chemicals.

You Can Prevent Adverse Health Effects

A powerful reason for optimism is that almost all of the adverse health effects caused by environmental hazards are preventable. When we take effective steps to eliminate or significantly reduce environmental hazards, the health benefits can be immediate, tangible, and dramatic. The elimination of leaded gasoline in Canada, the U.S., Australia, and many other nations lowered concentrations of lead in the air by more than 90%, causing a major decline in children's blood lead levels.

A global ban on the dirty dozen—twelve persistent organic pollutants including PCBs, dioxins, and several pesticides—has lowered people's body burdens of these chemicals, preventing countless cases of cancer, other debilitating illnesses, and premature deaths.

By reducing, or better yet eliminating, your exposures to harmful substances, you can decrease the risk of adverse health effects

For every toxic substance, process, or product in use today there is a safer alternative—either already in existence, or waiting to be discovered through the application of human intellect, ingenuity, and effort. In almost every case, the safer alternative is available at a comparable cost. Industry may reject these facts and fulminate about the high cost of acting, but history sets the record straight. The chemical industry denied that there were viable alternatives to ozone-depleting chemicals, predicting not only economic disaster but numerous deaths because food and vaccines would spoil without refrigeration. They were wrong. The motor vehicle industry initially denied that cars caused air pollution, then claimed that no technology existed to reduce pollution from vehicles, and later argued that installing devices to reduce air pollution would make cars prohibitively expensive. They were wrong every time. The pesticide industry argues that synthetic pesticides are absolutely necessary to grow food. Thousands of organic farmers are proving them wrong.

Nations that are acting to protect people from environmental hazards are not only global leaders in environmental protection but in public health, economic competitiveness, innovation, and happiness. They are proving that a greener, cleaner, healthier future is possible. Sweden is consistently at or near the top in international rankings of performance in protecting the environment and achieving good health. For decades the Swedes have been using strong public policies—enacting stringent regulations, shifting taxes from income and investment to pollution and waste, and investing in green technologies—to clean up their environment. Sweden also enjoys one of the world's most highly regarded health care systems, yet Swedish expenditures on health care have grown more slowly than any other wealthy industrialized nation over the past thirty years. This fact can be attributed partly to the country's strong environmental policies.

While progress is possible through stronger public policies and changes in business practices, individual actions can also make a huge difference in the level of environmental risks you face. By reducing, or better yet eliminating, your exposures to harmful substances, you can decrease the risk of adverse health effects. In one study, researchers tested the saliva and urine of children who switched from a conventional diet to a diet consisting entirely of organic food. When eating foods grown with pesticides, the children's urine and saliva contained biological markers of two organophosphates (malathion and chlorpyrifos), a group of pesticides derived from nerve gases used in World War II. When the children switched to an organic diet, all traces of pesticides in their bodies disappeared within eight to thirty-six hours. Similarly in the U.K., a study demonstrated that children whose diet was altered to exclude artificial food colors and preservatives were less likely to suffer from attention deficit hyperactivity disorder. In California and Canada, rates of lung cancer are falling as more and more people choose not to smoke. While there are obviously some factors beyond an individual's control, smart choices can greatly improve your health and likelihood of long life. Primarily, you can protect your health by:

> Identifying hazards.

> Eliminating sources of hazards.

> Limiting your exposure.

How This Book Can Help

This book contains the best scientific advice on minimizing the risks posed to your health by environmental hazards encountered in the air you breathe, both outdoors (Chapter 2) and indoors (Chapter 3), the food you eat (Chapter 4), the water you drink (Chapter 5), the consumer products you buy (Chapter 6), and the physical hazards you face (Chapter 7). While there are many simple and effective steps you can take to safeguard your health, certain risks are better addressed by governments and businesses—something you can ensure by exercising your powers as both a citizen and a consumer to influence public policy and corporate behavior (Chapter 8). As well, this book suggests how you can act to reduce the health risks associated with climate change and the decline of biological diversity, and how you can benefit from Nature's positive influences on your health (Chapter 9). Woven throughout the book you will find sidebars on various topics, including several that summarize our understanding of the connection between the environment and specific health concerns, including cancer and reproductive problems. In each chapter you will also find advice about those most vulnerable to environmental hazards—children—along with a checklist of actions you can take to protect yourself and your family.

The advice in this book for reducing or eliminating risks to your health caused by environmental factors is subject to three important caveats. The first caveat is that environmental risks to human health need to be evaluated in the context of other risk factors. For example, if you smoke tobacco, drink alcohol excessively, use illegal drugs, or are overweight or obese, it is almost certain that these factors pose a more substantial risk to your health than environmental hazards. It is illogical to worry about getting cancer from polluted air, contaminated food and water, or unsafe consumer products if you smoke a pack of cigarettes a day. Similarly, there is little point in fretting about pesticide residues on your produce if you eat an unhealthy diet or rarely participate in physical activities.

The second caveat is that there are some environmental risks individuals cannot completely avoid because either the hazards are ubiquitous (e.g., persistent organic pollutants) or information is not available for making sound decisions to reduce your risk. For example, in Australia, Canada, and all American states except California, laws fail to require the disclosure of toxic ingredients on most product labels. Cancer-causing chemicals can still be found in a wide range of everyday household products ranging from cosmetics to bathroom cleaners.

The third caveat is that the science of environmental health is evolving rapidly. New studies published during just one week in 2009 reported that:

- Men exposed to low levels of cadmium face an elevated risk of death from cancer and heart disease.

- Children living in homes where their parents use pesticides are twice as likely to develop brain cancer compared to children living in residences where no pesticides are used.

- Mice exposed to perfluorinated chemicals, which are used in the lining of food containers and in clothing, carpeting, upholstery, floor and car waxes, and firefighting foams, demonstrated "deranged spontaneous behavior" caused by changes in brain chemistry.

- The testosterone levels of men living in homes with high concentrations of flame retardants were significantly lower than the levels in men living in homes with low concentrations of these chemicals.

Although it is challenging to keep abreast of all of the information needed to protect our health, certain patterns have emerged. We often learn that substances previously believed to be benign are in fact harmful. We rarely discover that hazards once deemed harmful are in fact safe. It often turns out that substances once regarded as safe at certain levels of exposure are in fact dangerous at much lower levels. Lead is a classic example of this pattern. Health authorities have repeatedly lowered so-called acceptable levels of lead in our bodies. In the 1950s, blood lead levels above 60 micrograms per deciliter (μg/dl) were considered elevated. The blood lead level deemed elevated was then dropped to 40 μg/dl. Later it was lowered to 30 μg/dl and 25 μg/ dl. Today the maximum acceptable level is 10 μg/dl, but there is compelling evidence that adverse health effects occur below this, and many scientists believe that there is no safe level of exposure to lead. Another example is the regulatory limit for exposure to ben-

We rarely discover that hazards once deemed harmful are in fact safe

zene, a known carcinogen. The limit was first set in 1946 at 100 parts per million (ppm), lowered to 35 ppm, dropped to 25 ppm, lowered again to 10 ppm, and currently is set at 0.5 ppm. In other words, today's so-called safe level of benzene is less than 1% of what it was sixty years ago. Again, experts now believe there is no safe level of exposure to this potent carcinogen.

Key Concepts

Understanding a few key environmental health concepts will help make this book more useful for you. What do we mean by environmental hazards? Where do they come from? How are we exposed to them? How do we determine which hazards ought to be priorities for avoidance or reduction? Are some people more vulnerable than others?

Categories of Environmental Hazards

Environmental hazards fall into three categories—chemical, biological, and physical. Chemical hazards include pesticides, heavy metals, the air pollutants that make up smog, and the vast number of toxic substances produced by industry. Biological hazards include mold, dust mites, microorganisms that cause vector-borne diseases (e.g., West Nile enceph-alitis, Lyme disease), and the bacteria, protozoa, and viruses sometimes found in drinking water and food. Physical hazards include noise, extreme temperatures (both hot and cold), and all types of radiation (from the sun, x-rays, nuclear power plants, electric power lines, and other sources). Although this book focuses on chemical, biological, and physical hazards, it also addresses the indirect causes of harm to human health arising from poor urban design, climate change, ozone depletion, and the loss of biological diversity.

Sources

Knowing where environmental hazards come from will help you avoid them. Some environmental threats to human health occur naturally. Examples include radon, a radioactive gas that is found in the air of some buildings at dangerously high levels, and *Cryptosporidium*, a parasite that can contaminate drinking water supplies. Despite these natural hazards, there is little doubt that the majority of environmental threats to our health and well-being are the result of human activities. The twentieth century saw an unprecedented explosion in the manufacture, use, and release of chemicals. It is estimated that more than one hundred thousand chemicals are now produced in commercial volumes. Pollutant release inventories compiled by governments chronicle the release of trillions of kilograms of toxic substances into the air, water, soil, and ecosystems of industrialized nations each year, including carcinogens and chemicals that cause birth defects and developmental or reproductive problems. As well, humans have extracted substances such as lead, arsenic, mercury, uranium, and fossil fuels from the Earth's crust and released these substances and by-products from their use into ecosystems in quantities far exceeding natural background levels.

Many kitchens, laundry rooms, workshops, and medicine shelves hold dozens of harmful chemicals that may end up in the environment by way of sewers and landfills

Agricultural runoff (containing pesticides, fertilizers, antibiotics, hormones, and manure) and urban runoff (containing motor oil, animal waste, and pesticides) release billions of additional kilograms of toxic substances into our environment. Motor vehicles, driven trillions of kilometers each year, spew out billions of kilograms of health-harming emissions. Smaller sources of pollution, from gas stations to drycleaners, add to the total. Many kitchens, laundry rooms, workshops, and medicine shelves hold dozens of harmful chemicals that may end up in the environment by way of sewers and landfills. Perhaps most surprisingly, consumer products—air fresheners, baby toys, cosmetics, clothing, nonstick frying pans, vinyl products, furniture, and more—are sources of environmental hazards.

Despite its huge size, all parts of our world are interconnected. As a result, contaminants also reach us from far beyond our borders. The mercury contaminating Alaskan fish and as much as 15% of the particulate air pollution in western North America come from East Asia. Dangerous pesticides and other toxic chemicals, banned long ago in Canada, the U.S., and Europe but still used in developing nations, find their way here, traveling along air currents, moving through the water cycle, accumulating in food systems, or embedded in cheap products that we import. Asbestos, lead, and gamma-hydroxybutyrate (known as the date rape drug) have been found recently in children's toys imported from China.

Other risks arise from pollution that occurred years or even decades ago. Scattered across the landscape are tens of thousands of contaminated sites, including underground storage tanks that discharge petroleum products, obsolescent chemical plants, abandoned mines, leaking landfills, and illegal waste dumps. The threats to public health vary from site to site, from negligible to severe. For example, communities living near hazardous waste sites in the Great Lakes region of North America experience elevated levels of infant mortality, premature births, low birth weights, and cancer.

Exposure Routes
You can be exposed to chemical and biological hazards in five ways:

1. By inhaling air, both indoors and outdoors.
2. By consuming food, water, other beverages, and breast milk.

3. By direct contact with your skin (e.g., spilling pesticide on your hand).

4. By injection (e.g., being stung by a mosquito).

5. By exposure in utero (e.g., coming into contact with a chemical while in the womb—the developing fetus is exquisitely sensitive).

Knowing the main routes of exposure for specific environmental hazards will help you take effective steps to protect your health and the health of your children.

Determining Priorities

The degree of risk you face from a particular environmental hazard is determined by two main factors—the potency or toxicity of the hazard and the extent of your exposure. Almost any substance can be toxic at high enough levels. For example, drinking excess amounts of water can cause a condition called hyponatremia, which occasionally results in death. Some chemicals are so toxic that they can have adverse effects on human health when measured in parts per million or parts per billion (e.g., arsenic in drinking water). New scientific evidence suggests that some chemicals—particularly endocrine-disrupting chemicals—may actually be more toxic to humans at low levels than at high levels, challenging the conventional wisdom that "the dose makes the poison"—that higher doses are *always* more harmful. While the toxicity of environmental chemicals varies widely from substance to substance, we know little about the health effects of exposure to combinations of chemicals. In one recent experiment, scientists exposed tadpoles to a mixture of ten pesticides, all at levels well below what government and industry claim is safe. Ninety-nine percent of the tadpoles were killed.

While the toxicity of environmental chemicals varies widely from substance to substance, we know little about the health effects of exposure to combinations of chemicals

Exposure is the other half of the risk equation. For most environmental hazards, if you are not exposed at a high concentration, and not exposed often or for long, then you probably have nothing to worry about. For example, although asbestos is highly toxic, few members of the general public in the U.S., Canada, or Australia are likely to be exposed to asbestos at levels or for periods of time sufficient to endanger their health. Whether you wish to respond to a particular risk is an individual decision. The approach taken in this book is that if a hazard has low toxicity and there is a low likelihood of exposure, then it should generally be of low concern. Some people may still choose to take preventive action even though the risks appear to be low. Hazards that are highly toxic and involve a high likelihood of exposure should be top priorities for action to eliminate or reduce the risk.

Protecting the Vulnerable

Individuals and communities have different levels of susceptibility to environmental health impacts. Groups that face higher risks to their health from environmental hazards include members of certain ethnic groups, people living in poverty, individuals with compromised immune systems, children, and the elderly. Extensive research in the U.S. proves that African Americans, Hispanic Americans, Native Americans, and poor people generally bear a disproportionate burden of exposure to urban air pollution, hazardous waste sites, landfills, chemical plants, and other environmental health hazards. In part this is because marginalized groups lack political power, and in part because underprivileged people often end up living in the lower-cost housing that is available near polluting facilities. In Canada and Australia, Aboriginal people have suffered systemic environmental injustice, resulting in a devastating history of problems ranging from exposure to radioactive waste to the contamination of traditional foods with mercury, PCBs, and other pollutants.

Children are particularly vulnerable to environmental hazards for several reasons:

• Their behavior, diet, and physiology make them more likely than adults to experience higher levels of exposure (e.g., a 10-kilogram toddler may be more affected by exposure to the pesticide in an apple than a 50-kilogram adult).

- Their movement through key stages of development puts them at greater risk of being adversely affected by environmental exposures (e.g., a child exposed to mercury when her language or visual-spatial skills are developing may end up with learning difficulties).

- Their natural ability to defend against environmental harms is less developed (e.g., a child cannot metabolize some toxic substances into harmless ones the way an adult can).

- Their lives are just beginning, so they will be exposed to environmental chemicals for a longer period.

These factors often interact. Take exposure to lead for example. Young children spend more time outside and on the ground, and often place objects in their mouths. This means they are more likely to ingest lead in house dust, paint chips, and soil. Children also absorb a larger proportion of lead into their bodies than adults, and are vulnerable to lead's potentially devastating effects on their developing brains. All of these differences make children extremely vulnerable to the adverse neurological effects of lead. Other important environmental threats to the health of children are indoor air quality, outdoor air quality, water contaminants, environmental tobacco smoke, mercury, and pesticides. If we can create an environment that is safe and healthy for children, the most sensitive and vulnerable among us, we will create an environment safe and healthy for all.

Certain individuals may also face elevated health risks because of their genetic characteristics (see page 27). A familiar illustration of this is the way different people respond to bee stings. For most of us, a bee sting is a painful but fleeting experience that poses no serious danger. For one or two people in a thousand, however, genetic differences mean that a single bee sting can cause a life-threatening reaction called anaphylaxis, a severe allergic response. Individuals can also have variations in the genes that govern how we metabolize toxic substances, so that certain chemicals harmless to most people can make them sick. Some individuals are ten thousand times more sensitive to certain types of air pollution. It is estimated that one in forty people suffers from some form of chemical sensitivity, increasing their vulnerability to pollution. Even if a small proportion of people (e.g., 1% to 5%) have a genetic variation that increases their vulnerability to a specific environmental hazard, this can still translate into hundreds of thousands of affected people in Canada or Australia and millions of affected people in the U.S. or Europe. As Professor Judith Stern from the University of California, Davis observes, "genetics loads the gun, but the environment pulls the trigger."

Some individuals are ten thousand times more sensitive to certain types of air pollution

Guiding Principles

At the heart of this book are three fundamental principles for dodging the toxic bullet. First, every person has the right to breathe clean air, drink clean water, and live in a healthy environment. The right to live in a healthy environment is critical; without this, all other human rights lose their meaning. The constitutions of more than eighty nations (not including Canada, the U.S., or Australia), as well as international agreements covering Europe, Latin America, the Middle East, and Africa, provide legal recognition of the right to a healthy environment. There is a catch, however, that is often overlooked in societies where individual rights are predominant, and the catch is that with rights come responsibilities. The responsibility that accompanies your right to live in a healthy environment is the duty to do everything in your power to protect the beauty, diversity, and health of the planet.

The precautionary principle is the second basic tenet of this book. This means that when we have some scientific evidence that a substance or activity is harming human health or the environment, a lack of certainty must not be used to block action to address the harm. To most people this makes perfect sense—it's better to be safe than sorry. And yet as a society, despite the catastrophic impacts of PCBs, CFCs, DDT, and other toxic chemicals, we still have not learned this basic lesson. Our ongoing folly is illustrated by polybrominated diphenyl ethers (PBDEs), a group of chemicals widely used as flame retardants. PBDEs are toxic to the brain, liver, thyroid, and reproductive and immune systems, and they may cause cancer. In the 1990s, scientists discovered that PBDEs were rapidly accumulating in the breast milk of mothers from Sweden to Canada and Japan. PBDEs were also turning up in wildlife, from polar bears and killer whales to peregrine falcons and wild salmon. Once it was discovered that these compounds were building up in people's bodies, PBDE manufacturing and use should have been immediately suspended until industry provided reliable scientific evidence that these substances did not threaten either human health or the environment. No such global action was taken. Eventually, European governments, led by Sweden and Norway, banned these substances, and Canada and several American states followed with partial bans. Unfortunately, many nations, including the U.S. and Australia, still allow the use of PBDEs. North American children today have the highest body burden of these chemicals in the world, a situation that might have been avoided by applying the precautionary principle to PBDEs: instituting an immediate global ban and requiring the use of safer substitutes.

The right to live in a healthy environment is critical; without this, all other human rights lose their meaning

The third principle this book is founded upon is that an ounce of prevention is worth a pound of cure. This old folk saying does not translate well into metric (27 grams of prevention are worth 454 grams of cure) but has otherwise stood the test of time. There is a mountain of evidence proving beyond any reasonable doubt that it's more effective and less expensive to prevent pollution than to attempt to clean up the mess after the fact, considering the colossal costs of human suffering and

>> YOUR EXPOSURE TO TOXIC SUBSTANCES
MAY HARM YOUR GRANDCHILDREN

A FEW YEARS AGO, scientists believed that the Human Genome Project, which mapped roughly twenty-five thousand human genes, would be a silver bullet for curing disease. Although some promising steps forward have been taken, the relationship between our genes and disease is more complex than anticipated. Epigenetics is the science of how genes behave (or express themselves), and is to genetics what software is to computer hardware. New research in epigenetics has identified multigenerational effects of exposure to toxic substances that operate not through genetic mutation but through a more subtle process called methylation, changing the way genes behave. Genes may be switched on or off by toxic exposures, increasing vulnerability to specific diseases and disorders. In genetic terms, if an individual has two tumor-suppressing genes, but one gene is turned off and the other breaks down, that individual is more susceptible to cancer. This is like flying a two-engine airplane with one engine off. If the second engine quits, the plane is much more likely to crash.

In several experiments exploring the effects of hormone-disrupting chemicals, scientists exposed pregnant rats to extremely low doses of bisphenol A, a substance widely used in plastic products. The prenatal exposure resulted in higher risks of prostate and breast cancer among the rats' offspring. Similarly, when pregnant mice were exposed to vinclozolin (a pesticide known to disrupt the endocrine system), four generations of male offspring experienced reduced sperm production. These discoveries suggest that direct exposure is not necessary to cause harm, meaning that your exposure to a toxic substance could negatively affect the health of your grandchildren, and that your grandchildren could pass on the problem originating with your exposure to their children.

environmental damage. Regulations enacted in Canada, the U.S., and Australia to reduce various air pollutants have cost billions of dollars but have also generated trillions in benefits. Stronger regulations would have higher costs but would produce even greater benefits. Ensuring clean air—by reducing air pollution in industrialized nations to preindustrial levels—would add almost an additional year to everyone's life expectancy. Eliminating mercury exposure in the U.S., and preventing the IQ loss that can result, would save an estimated US$8.7 billion annually in diminished economic productivity (US$2.2 billion to US$43.8 billion). Protecting human health from environmental hazards is a smart investment.

Wrap-up

Nine out of ten people today are worried about the impacts of air pollution, contaminated food and water, unsafe consumer products, and climate change on their health and their children's health. These concerns are understandable, given the magnitude of today's environmental problems. Yet it is also important to recognize that there is no such thing as a perfectly safe environment. The world is and always will be full of risks, but we can eliminate and reduce unnecessary and preventable risks. Knowledge is a powerful antidote to fear. This book empowers you with the information needed to make wise choices and create a cleaner, greener, healthier lifestyle.

Taking steps to reduce the environmental threats to your health will generate a host of other benefits. Your actions can make the air and water cleaner for everyone; improve working conditions in factories, farms, and other occupational settings; protect Nature and biodiversity; and reduce the threats posed by climate change. Your ecological footprint (a measure of your total environmental impact) will shrink, not only taking pressure off the planet but also increasing the likelihood that you will lead a happy and fulfilling life.

2 THE OUTDOOR AIR WE BREATHE

I'm so old, I can remember when the air was clean and sex was dirty.

George Burns

IT'S NO SECRET that air is fundamental to human life. We breathe in
an estimated 15,000 liters (almost 4,000 gallons) of air daily, approximately 10 liters every minute. Every time we inhale, we draw air across
55 to 85 square meters (600 to 900 square feet) of surface area in our
alveoli, tiny sacs inside the lungs. Life-giving oxygen immediately passes
into our bloodstream. Twenty-five trillion red blood cells, each containing 300 million hemoglobin molecules, transport oxygen from the lungs
to the heart and around our bodies. Carbon dioxide is simultaneously
returned to the lungs and exhaled. All of the blood in our system does a
complete lap per minute when we are resting, and as many as five laps per
minute during intense exercise.

In 2008, a remarkable world record for unassisted breath-holding
was set by Germany's Tom Sietas, who held his breath for ten minutes
and twelve seconds. In 2009, a world record for assisted breath-holding
was set by David Merlini, who held his breath for more than twenty minutes while submerged in a tank full of water at a Formula 1 auto race in
Bahrain. He gained an edge by breathing pure oxygen for half an hour
before his stunt, thus super-oxygenating his blood. Unlike Sietas and

Merlini, most people will pass out after being deprived of oxygen for two or three minutes. After a brief period of unconsciousness, the heart will stop pumping. Within minutes, electrical activity in the brain will come to a halt because neurons are deprived of oxygen. This is the modern definition of biological death.

Given the importance of air to human life and well-being, it is incredible how cavalier we are about using the atmosphere as a gigantic trash can. The word smog (a mash-up of smoke and fog) dates back to the beginning of the twentieth century. The timing is no coincidence, as this is when motor vehicles started hitting the streets and fossil fuel-powered industrialization shifted into high gear. The dominant sources of air pollution today are industrial facilities (led by coal-fired power plants, metal smelters, pulp and paper mills, petroleum refineries, and chemical factories), mobile sources (diesel trucks, heavy-duty vehicles, SUVs, cars, motorcycles, trains, boats, and planes), agriculture, and residential burning of fossil fuels and wood. Consumer products ranging from leaf-blowers to gas lawn mowers and Jet Skis also emit a small but growing share of air pollution. Industrial facilities in the U.S., Canada, and Australia spew billions of tonnes of pollutants (trillions of kilograms!) into the atmosphere annually, including known or suspected carcinogens, such as styrene, benzene, and formaldehyde.

Many of the same toxic substances found in tobacco smoke are present in vehicle exhaust

In 1950, there were about 50 million cars in the world. Today there are almost that many vehicles in California alone, while the global total is speeding toward one billion. Vehicles now outnumber drivers in the U.S., and Americans drive more than 8 trillion kilometers (5 trillion miles) annually as a result of living in sprawling urban communities (see page 36). Although individual cars emit less pollution today than in the past, the sheer number of cars and the distance they are driven overwhelm technological progress. Vehicle exhaust is a nasty stew of toxic substances, including sulfur dioxide, nitrogen oxides, particulate matter, and carbon monoxide, as well as thousands of hazardous air pollutants. Many of the same toxic substances found in tobacco smoke are present in vehicle exhaust, including benzene, polycyclic aromatic hydrocarbons (PAHs), 1,3-butadiene, formaldehyde, acrolein, heavy metals, and hexane. This is one reason health experts compare living in some cities to smoking a pack of cigarettes daily.

Burning wood may seem like a benign, even environmentally friendly alternative to fossil fuels. To the contrary, woodstoves, fireplaces, and wood boilers are major sources of both outdoor and indoor air pollution. Burning wood produces high levels of particulate pollution as well as carbon monoxide, nitrogen dioxide, sulfur dioxide, hydrochloric acid, formaldehyde, and PAHs. Outdoor PAH levels in residential areas during winter can reach levels comparable to PAH concentrations in second-hand tobacco smoke.

Some types of air pollution (e.g., sulfur dioxide emissions, which cause acid rain, and lead emissions from gasoline) have decreased in recent decades. We are no longer plagued by catastrophes such as the lethal London smog of 1952 that killed as many as 12,000 people in a short span of time, causing undertakers to run out of caskets. Decreases in air pollution cause direct and immediate health benefits. When Dublin, Ireland, banned the residential burning of coal, deaths caused by respiratory illness fell 15% and heart disease fell by 10%. During the 1996 Summer Olympic Games in Atlanta, restrictions on vehicle traffic caused a decrease in ozone levels and a corresponding decrease in children suffering asthma attacks. When Hong Kong passed a law restricting the amount of sulfur in gasoline, the number of deaths caused by respiratory and heart disease fell.

Despite progress in reducing levels of some air pollutants, there are still more than 185 million Americans living in areas that fail to meet federal ozone and particulate pollution standards. Six out of ten Americans live in counties where ozone levels place them at risk for decreased lung function, respiratory infections, and aggravation of respiratory illness. Three out of ten Americans live in areas where short-term spikes in fine particle pollution raise their risks of asthma attacks, heart attacks, strokes, and early death. Similarly, the majority of Canadians are exposed to smog at concentrations that pose a threat to their health.

Major Outdoor Air Pollutants

Air pollution involves many compounds that harm our health: microscopic airborne particles, ozone, sulfur dioxide, nitrogen oxides, carbon monoxide, volatile organic compounds, and other hazardous pollutants.

Particulate Matter

Particulate matter, also known as particle pollution, is composed of microscopic dust or liquid droplets suspended in the air. Particles are classified according to size. Fine and ultrafine particles less than 2.5 microns in size (one-thirtieth the width of a human hair) are more likely to penetrate deep into the lungs, harming your health. Fine particulate matter is created by the combustion of fossil fuels (coal, oil, natural gas, gasoline, diesel fuel) required in the petroleum, cement, lumber, pulp, and mining industries as well as in transportation. Coarse particulate matter originates from road dust, diesel engines, smelting, demolition, and crushing and grinding operations. Residential wood burning, forest fires, windblown soil, pollens, molds, volcanic emissions, and sea spray can also produce particle pollution.

Temporary symptoms from exposure to elevated levels of particles include eye, nose, and throat irritation; coughing; phlegm production; chest tightness; and shortness of breath. Particle pollution is also linked to impaired development of children's lungs, increased numbers of asthma attacks, chronic bronchitis, heart attacks, strokes, lung cancer, and early deaths from respiratory and cardiovascular diseases. There is no safe level of fine particulate matter. Some people will experience negative health effects even at low levels, and the proportion of people affected will rise as levels of particle pollution increase.

Ozone

Ozone, a key element in smog, is formed by atmospheric reactions involving nitrogen oxides, volatile organic compounds, and sunlight. Humans contribute to this process mainly by burning fossil fuels, which leads to the production of nitrogen oxides and volatile organic compounds. Sunlight intensity and higher temperatures exacerbate the formation of ozone, explaining why smog is generally worse during summer months and from midday through the afternoon. Ozone can travel long distances, affecting rural areas downwind from cities.

> Sunlight intensity and higher temperatures exacerbate the formation of ozone, explaining why smog is generally worse during summer months and from midday through the afternoon

Ozone irritates the respiratory tract. Think of it as sunburn on your lungs. Exposure to ozone can cause shortness of breath, chest pain, coughing, wheezing, increased susceptibility to respiratory infections, and increased risk of asthma attacks. Ozone contributes to increased hospital admissions for acute respiratory conditions such as chronic obstructive pulmonary disease, and increases the risk of premature death. There is no safe level of ozone. Ground-level ozone must be distinguished from stratospheric ozone, which provides the vital service of blocking harmful ultraviolet radiation from the sun.

Sulfur Dioxide

Most sulfur dioxide emissions are produced by the production, processing, and combustion of fossil fuels, as well as by metal smelting and refining. Exposure to sulfur dioxide can cause severe problems for people with asthma and is linked to increased risks of lung cancer and chronic bronchitis. Sulfur dioxide also reacts with other air pollutants to form particulate matter.

Nitrogen Oxides

Nitrogen oxides are odorless gases produced by the combustion of fossil fuels. Exposure to elevated levels of nitrogen oxides can contribute to eye, nose, and throat irritation, shortness of breath, respiratory illness, aggravation of asthma, decreased lung function, increased risk of respiratory infection, and reduced lung growth in children. Nitrogen oxides react with oxygen to form ozone, and with other air pollutants to form smog.

Carbon Monoxide

Carbon monoxide is an invisible, odorless gas produced by the incomplete combustion of fossil fuels, largely from motor vehicles, residential wood burning, and industry. When inhaled, carbon monoxide interferes with the blood's ability to deliver oxygen throughout the body. At high concentrations it can cause unconsciousness and death. Lower concentrations can adversely affect the functioning of the heart and cause headaches, dizziness, weakness, nausea, confusion, fatigue, low birth weight, and preterm births. However, outdoor concentrations of carbon monoxide rarely reach dangerous levels.

Volatile Organic Compounds

Volatile organic compounds (VOCs) are chemicals containing carbon that easily evaporate and form gases or vapors at room temperature. VOCs are produced by the use of fossil fuels in transportation, petroleum production and processing, and industrial applications. Residential wood burning also releases VOCs, as do many solvents, adhesives, paints and stains, building materials, and other consumer products. VOCs such as benzene, toluene, ethylbenzene, and xylene are linked to eye irritation, headaches, breathing problems, impaired brain development, and cancer.

Hazardous Air Pollutants

There are hundreds of other air pollutants that are known or suspected to cause cancer, genetic mutation, and birth defects, even at relatively low exposure levels. Hazardous air pollutants are released by motor vehicles, factories, and incinerators. Examples include mercury, which is associated with developmental deficits in children, and polycyclic aromatic hydrocarbons, which cause cancer. The U.S. Environmental Protection Agency estimates that the cancer risk from hazardous air pollutants is fifty times higher than the level governments usually deem acceptable. Some of these pollutants, such as PCBs, mercury, and dioxins, may be released in one geographic area and spread across a continent or around the world.

The Adverse Health Effects of Air Pollution

Exposure to air pollution can cause a host of symptoms—shortness of breath, wheezing, headaches, eye irritation—and cause or contribute to asthma attacks, emphysema, bronchitis, chronic obstructive pulmonary disease, deep vein thrombosis, heart disease, stroke, cancer, neuro-degenerative disease, and premature death. Air pollution's adverse effects on our health can begin even before we are born, contributing to mis-carriage, preterm delivery, and lower birth weight (see page 39). Pregnant women in Los Angeles exposed to higher levels of smog suffer triple the risk of birth defects such as defective heart valves and cleft lips and palates.

Air pollution may be the deadliest environmen-tal problem facing people who live in industrialized nations, killing hundreds of thousands of people annually. The Canadian Medical Association esti-mates that twenty-one thousand premature deaths occur in Canada annually as a result of exposure to air pollution, while the figure for the U.S., where cities endure smoggier air, could be up to ten times that. Experts estimate that individuals living in the smoggiest American and Canadian cities lose between 1.8 and 3.1 years of life expectancy because of long-term exposure to air pollution.

Twenty-one thousand premature deaths occur in Canada annually as a result of exposure to air pollution

The main cause of death associated with exposure to air pollution is heart disease. Microscopic particles of air pollution are inhaled deep into the lungs, where they can enter the bloodstream and trigger a cascade of

URBAN SPRAWL «

FOR THE FIRST time, more people live in cities than in rural communities. In Canada, the U.S., and Australia, most people are now urbanites. For the past century, urban planning has reflected the values of our car culture, with sprawling suburban housing and a proliferation of roads and freeways. This kind of urban design has made public transit unworkable, reduced opportunities for walking and cycling, and encouraged the sedentary habits now contributing to an obesity epidemic. Sprawl has also caused air pollution, water contamination, the loss of natural habitat and farmland, and an erosion of social capital while contributing to five vexing health problems—cardiovascular disease, cancer, lung disease, motor vehicle injuries, and depression.

Fortunately, there is a better way to build cities. Compact urban design and Smart Growth, with plentiful public green space, as employed in places like Amsterdam, Copenhagen, and Vancouver, encourage walking and cycling, facilitate public transit, and improve social cohesion, a key element of happiness. The residents of Copenhagen, one of the world's most bicycle-friendly cities, cycle for 36% of all their trips. By 2015, Copenhagen aims to increase this figure to 50%, with health and economic benefits that include preventing forty-six thousand years of prolonged illness and saving over US$40 million in health care costs and lost productivity.

In Stockholm, another example of Smart Growth, more than 90% of residents live within 300 meters (roughly 300 yards) of a public park or other green space. Making cities healthier and more livable also provides environmental benefits, such as cleaner air, lower greenhouse gas emissions, and more habitat where Nature can flourish.

physiological responses in the cardiovascular system, including inflammation, changes in the composition of the blood, increased propensity to form clots, hardening and narrowing of the arteries, and abnormal heartbeat. For example, exposure to diesel fumes contributes to the formation of blood clots, which can lead to heart attacks and strokes. Similarly, air pollution is implicated in some cases of deep vein thrombosis, a serious ailment in which a blood clot forms in the deep leg vein, causing damage to the leg and creating the risk of a life-threatening pulmonary embolism (where the clot is transported through the circulatory system, becomes trapped in the lung, blocks the oxygen supply, and causes heart failure).

Heart disease is the leading cause of death in the U.S., Canada, and Australia. And while each person's increased risk because of air pollution is small when compared with increased risk because of smoking, obesity, or high blood pressure, the number of people exposed to unhealthy levels of air pollution is so great—hundreds of millions—that the impact in terms of total illnesses and premature deaths is substantial.

Who Is Vulnerable

We are all vulnerable to the adverse health effects of air pollution. Your reaction to air pollutants will depend on:

- The types of pollutants you are exposed to.
- Your age and stage of development.
- Your overall health.
- Your genetic makeup.
- The amount and duration of your exposure.

Even healthy people who are exposed to air pollution may experience irritated eyes, coughing, increased mucus production, and breathing difficulties, especially during exercise or other strenuous activities. However, some people are particularly susceptible to air pollution, including those already suffering from respiratory or cardiovascular disease, young children, and the elderly.

Because air pollution makes it harder to breathe, anyone with a respiratory illness (chronic obstructive pulmonary disease, bronchitis, emphysema, asthma), or a heart condition (angina, previous heart attack, congestive heart failure, irregular heartbeat) is sensitive to air pollution. Individuals with lung or heart disease may experience increased frequency and/or severity of symptoms, and increased medication requirements. People with respiratory illnesses may notice an increase in coughing wheezing, shortness of breath, or phlegm. Individuals with heart problems may feel light-headed and experience increased shortness of breath, arm or chest pain, fluttering in the chest, and swelling in the ankles and feet. You can have lung or heart disease and not know it. Anyone experiencing one of the following symptoms during or after outdoor activities—pain, tightness or fluttering in the chest, difficulty breathing without considerable exertion, persistent cough or shortness of breath, or a light-headed feeling—should consult a doctor.

Exposure to air pollution at an early age can impair lung development and cause permanent damage to the respiratory system

Children and the elderly are especially vulnerable to air pollution. Relative to their size, children breathe more air than adults, their airways are narrower and more susceptible to irritation, and their natural defense systems are not fully developed. Children also spend more time outside than adults and engage in more vigorous activities. Exposure to air pollution at an early age can impair lung development and cause permanent damage to the respiratory system. Seniors are susceptible to air pollution because of weaker overall health, diminished functioning of their immune systems, and respiratory or cardiovascular conditions—some of which may be undiagnosed.

There is growing recognition that air pollution has a disproportionate impact on certain ethnic groups and low-income neighborhoods. For example, in the U.S., approximately 61% of African American children,

TOXIC CHEMICALS ARE contributing to reductions in fertility, alterations in sexual behavior, deformations of the reproductive tract, and reproductive diseases. Specific health outcomes linked to environmental factors are declining quantity and quality of sperm, difficulty becoming pregnant (delayed conception), spontaneous abortion, stillbirth, preterm birth, low birth weight, and birth defects. Some nations have witnessed an increase in the prevalence of several male genital birth defects, including hypospadias, where the opening of the urethra is on the underside rather than the tip of the penis. Endocrine-disrupting chemicals are prime suspects in this trend.

There has also been a statistically significant decline in the ratio of male to female births in several industrialized countries, including Canada, Germany, and the U.S. Perhaps the most extreme case involves the Aamjiwnaang First Nation, whose people live beside Sarnia, Ontario, near the U.S. border. The area is a notorious pollution hotspot, with more than sixty chemical and petrochemical plants nearby. Between 1999 and 2003 the proportion of male babies born to Aamjiwnaang women fell from normal levels (slightly more than 50%) to less than 35% of all births. Researchers believe exposure to environmental chemicals that affect the reproductive system may be a major factor. Evidence links dioxins, mercury, PCBs, and pesticides to changes in gender ratios.

As Dr. Stephen Genuis wrote in the journal *Reproductive Toxicology* in 2009, "Future generations of scientists will look back with disbelief at a medical culture that permitted poisoning of reproductive-aged women and ignored ramifications to unborn children."

See www.ourstolenfuture.org for additional information.

69% of Hispanic American children, and 68% of Asian American children live in areas with high ozone levels, while only 51% of white children live in such areas.

How to Protect Yourself and Others

Spending time outside and getting regular physical exercise are two vitally important elements of a healthy lifestyle. Because we have become sedentary and indoor-focused, most of us would benefit from spending more time being active outside, preferably in natural settings. This is particularly important to the health and development of children.

The most attractive seasons to spend time outside are the warmer seasons, which generally coincide with the worst air pollution. Unfortunately, working, playing, gardening, or exercising outside can make you vulnerable to the adverse effects of air pollution. Because your muscles need oxygen to function, you breathe more rapidly and inhale air deeper into your lungs when you are physically active. Strenuous activities can also cause you to breathe more through your mouth, which is a less effective pollution filter than your nose. Endurance athletes are acutely aware of the dangers posed by air pollution, because they breathe the greatest volumes of air while training and competing. World record-holder Haile Gebrselassie of Ethiopia skipped the marathon at the 2008 Summer Olympic Games in Beijing because of the city's notoriously polluted air.

So how can you protect yourself from air pollution? Above all, keep enjoying physical activities outdoors, but do so wisely by following these recommendations.

Be aware of the quality of the air you breathe. Most governments provide a daily air quality index rating that can help you decide how much time to spend outside and during what parts of the day:

Canada's Air Quality Health Index

LOW RISK	1–3—Enjoy your usual outdoor activities
MODERATE RISK	4–6—Vulnerable groups, such as people with heart or breathing problems, may reduce, relocate, or reschedule strenuous outdoor activities if they experience symptoms such as wheezing, coughing, or throat irritation
HIGH RISK	7–10—Vulnerable groups, such as people with heart or breathing problems, should reduce, relocate, or reschedule outdoor activities. Children and the elderly should also take it easy, while everyone else may reduce or reschedule strenuous outdoor activities if they experience symptoms such as wheezing, coughing, or throat irritation
VERY HIGH RISK	10+—Vulnerable groups, children, and the elderly should avoid strenuous activities outdoors. Everyone should reduce or reschedule strenuous activities outdoors, especially if you experience symptoms such as wheezing, coughing, or throat irritation

See www.airhealth.ca

Australia's Air Quality Index

VERY GOOD	0–33
GOOD	34–66
FAIR	67–99
POOR	100–149
VERY POOR	150 or greater

See www.epa.vic.gov.au

U.S. Environmental Protection Agency Air Quality Index

GOOD	0–50—Air pollution poses little or no short-term risk
MODERATE	51–100—For some pollutants there may be a moderate health concern for a small number of people
UNHEALTHY FOR SENSITIVE GROUPS	101–150—Members of sensitive groups (e.g., people with lung or heart disease) may experience adverse health effects
UNHEALTHY	151–200—Everyone may begin to experience adverse health effects
VERY UNHEALTHY	201–300—Health alert issued, everyone may experience more serious health effects
HAZARDOUS	301–500—Health warnings due to emergency conditions. The entire population is more likely to be affected

See www.airnow.gov

Throughout the world, media outlets report on air quality. When you learn from media reports or the Internet that air quality is particularly bad, you should defer outdoor activities for another time, find an alternative activity indoors, or limit the intensity and amount of time spent outside. If you experience any unusual coughing, chest discomfort, wheezing, or breathing difficulty, you should reduce your activity level immediately. If you have a heart or lung condition, talk to your doctor about additional ways to protect your health when air pollution levels are high.

When you learn from media reports or the Internet that air quality is particularly bad, you should defer outdoor activities for another time

It's also important to understand that the air quality index is intended to prevent short-term health problems such as asthma attacks and heart attacks. However, even when the index reports low risk, air pollution can still contribute to long-term health problems. Keep in mind that governments in Australia, Canada, and the U.S. set air quality standards at levels that are economically feasible (that is, they place considerable weight on the economic costs of reducing pollution) rather than at levels considered best for human health.

Schedule exercise, play, and other outdoor activities in the early morning or in the evening. Avoid outdoor activities in the middle of the day and the afternoon, except in winter. Smog tends to worsen later in the day because it is a product of sunlight, temperature, and ground-level ozone, which in turn is caused by emissions of nitrogen oxides and volatile organic compounds. Pollutants released by vehicles during the morning rush hour react and combine to make midday and early afternoon the worst times for air quality in most locations.

Avoid living, working, or playing in close proximity to roads with high traffic volumes or industrial facilities. To the extent that it is possible, choose homes, workplaces, and schools that are a healthy distance from major sources of air pollution, including busy roads and industrial facilities. Living within 500 meters (500 yards) of major roads can contribute to hardening of the arteries (raising the risk of heart disease and stroke), severely affect children's lung development (leading to decreased lung function later in life), and exacerbate asthma. Exposure to diesel exhaust, which contains a high volume of ultrafine particles, can also contribute to cancer. Nursing homes, daycare facilities, schools, and other places frequented by the elderly and children should always be located away from busy streets in order to protect these vulnerable people.

In any case, avoid exercise, play, and other outdoor activities near industrial areas, busy streets, or streets with heavy truck and bus traffic to avoid exposure to high volumes of diesel exhaust. A buffer of at least 200 meters, and ideally more than 500 meters, is recommended.

You can learn about industrial air pollution in your neighborhood (or a place where you are considering moving) at websites that organize pollution information geographically. In the U.S., go to www.scorecard.org and enter your zip code. In Canada, go to www.pollutionwatch.org and enter your postal code.

Choose green alternatives to driving. Alternatives to driving include walking, cycling, taking public transit, carpooling, joining a car-sharing co-op, and finding ways to travel less often—working four days a week or telecommuting. If you walk or cycle to work, find routes that minimize your exposure to vehicle traffic, such as a pathway that doesn't permit motorized traffic, or a series of quiet side streets. If there's no alternative to busy roads, consider purchasing high-quality personal protective equipment. A properly fitted mask with a HEPA (high-efficiency particulate air) filter can reduce inhalation of hydrocarbons, nitrogen oxides, sulfur dioxide, smoke, and fine particulates, and can make a political statement about the need to improve air quality in your community.

People traveling in cars as drivers or passengers are exposed to just as much air pollution as pedestrians or cyclists, and sometimes more. In Sydney, Australia, a group of volunteers participated in an experiment by traveling to work using different modes of transport—rail, bus, cycling, walking, and private vehicles. Car commuters had the highest exposure to volatile organic compounds while bus riders experienced the highest levels of nitrogen oxides. Cyclists, walkers, and train passengers were exposed to lower levels of these pollutants. Air quality inside a vehicle becomes significantly worse if there is traffic congestion, as is often the case during rush hour. Motorists are two to three times more likely to have heart attacks when stuck in traffic, and rate commuting as the worst part of their day. In contrast, people who walk or cycle to work not only get the heart and health benefits of exercise but also rate their commute as one of the highlights of their day.

If you walk or cycle to work, find routes that minimize your exposure to vehicle traffic

Drive a clean vehicle, and use it less. New vehicles are much cleaner than older models, and keeping engines tuned and tires inflated will save you money and reduce emissions. Planning ahead to do all of your errands in one trip instead of two or three will help reduce pollution.

Become a clean air advocate. You have the right to breathe clean air. In order to enjoy this right, you need to push governments at all levels, from local to national, to implement stronger clean air policies, including health-based air quality standards (especially for particle pollution and ozone); tax policies that discourage congestion and pollution; investment in infrastructure for walking, cycling, and other forms of nonmotorized transport; planning that creates more compact cities, lower speed limits; and switching subsidies from oil, gas, and coal to clean renewable forms of energy. Dirty power plants, particularly those that burn coal, should be mothballed as soon as possible. Stricter fuel-efficiency standards for vehicles are long overdue. Stronger regulations are especially important for diesel vehicles and for ships, which currently generate disproportionate amounts of pollution.

Projects at the local level often produce tangible results more quickly than larger-scale efforts. Consider contributing to traffic calming strategies in your neighborhood, participating in Bike to Work Week, and joining restoration or reforestation projects. In Canada, celebrate Clean

Air Day, held every June, by taking a new step to improve your community's air. This could be anything from a personal commitment to driving less to planting a tree to advocating for stronger clean air policies.

Avoid backyard burning. Backyard burning of scrap wood and trash is a major source of particle pollution and hazardous air pollutants. It is dangerous to burn garbage, plywood, painted wood, and other materials in woodstoves and fireplaces. These activities are particularly likely to harm you and your family because of harmful combustion by-products and high levels of exposure. It is especially dangerous to burn pressure-treated wood containing arsenic and chromium. Wood-burning backyard boilers have recently become popular for home heating and hot water but produce high volumes of smoke and particle pollution.

Protect yourself from wildfires. Wildfires are in the news more often these days. Higher temperatures, changes in precipitation patterns (both associated with climate change), the expansion of human settlements, and misguided forest management strategies are resulting in heightened risks of wildfires. These fires can generate staggering levels of air pollution, far in excess of what even the most polluted modern city would normally experience. Take special precautions if there are major fires near your community:

> Avoid inhaling smoke, ashes, soot, or particles.

> Stay indoors, keeping doors, windows, and fireplace dampers closed.

> Refrain from exercising outdoors if you can smell smoke or if your eyes or throat become irritated.

> Keep windows and vents closed when driving through smoky areas.

> If you must venture outdoors, breathe through a damp cloth to filter out some particulate pollution.

> Be particularly careful if you have lung or heart disease or asthma, as exposure to smoke can exacerbate symptoms.

> Seek medical attention if you experience pain or difficulty breathing, a persistent cough, or if your usual medications do not relieve respiratory symptoms.

> Be aware that ordinary dust masks do not offer adequate protection from the dangerous fine particles resulting from fires. Use an N95 respirator, a type of mask that can filter out harmful fine particles and be adjusted to fit tightly on the face.

Advice for Parents

Children are especially vulnerable to air pollution. Protect children's health by taking these steps:

> Pay attention to your local air quality index. When air quality is poor, children should play inside or avoid strenuous outdoor exercise.

> Keep children's outdoor activities as far as possible from busy roadways and other sources of pollution. A good rule of thumb for a minimum buffer is 500 meters (500 yards).

> Encourage your children and their friends to walk or bicycle to school. Walking school bus programs are growing in popularity throughout Canada, the U.S., and Australia. See www.walkingschoolbus.org for general information.

> Encourage your children's school to reduce school bus emissions. Many buses use older, heavily polluting diesel engines; newer engines are cleaner. Schools should not allow school buses to idle nearby. See www.epa.gov/cleanschoolbus for more on school buses.

> If your children have asthma, make sure they have inhalers with them at all times, and have a backup available at school or daycare. Consider using a MedicAlert bracelet to provide vital information to health care authorities in the event of an emergency.

> Be an advocate for your children's health. Make sure other parents, teachers, coaches, daycare operators, school administrators, and camp officials know about air pollution, respond to air quality ratings, and display other air-smart behavior.

Wrap-up

The staggering price we pay for air pollution includes direct health care costs, lost productivity, premature death costs, and the pain and suffering caused by nonfatal illnesses. In the U.S., air pollution costs up to US$670 billion annually. In one Canadian province alone (Ontario), the costs of air pollution are estimated to exceed Cdn$9 billion annually.

The devastating impacts on human health from air pollution could be almost entirely prevented if steps were taken to reduce emissions from power plants, factories, other businesses, and motor vehicles. Stronger laws and policies to reduce air pollution are urgently needed. Cost-benefit analyses of existing environmental laws mandating the elimination of lead from gasoline, reductions in sulfur dioxide emissions, and the phase-out of ozone-depleting substances prove that, contrary to industries' claims, the net economic impacts are positive rather than negative. From 1975 to 2000, air pollution regulations in the U.S. created benefits totalling $5.4 trillion while imposing costs of less than $1 trillion. Similarly, for every dollar invested in reducing pollution from diesel engines, society gains approximately $13 in health and environmental benefits.

Given the huge health benefits of both exercise and time spent outside in natural settings, it would be a public health disaster if people reduced these activities because of concerns about air pollution. Spend more time outside and participate in more physical activities, but do so wisely to maximize the health benefits. The advice in this chapter will help you breathe easier and result in a cleaner, healthier environment for everyone.

Breathe Clean Outdoor Air

> Keep an eye on the air quality index, especially during the summer.

> Schedule outdoor activities in the early morning or evening.

> Avoid living, playing, or exercising near industrial facilities or busy roads.

> Choose green alternatives to driving whenever possible.

> Drive a clean vehicle and use it less often.

> Become a clean-air advocate.

> Do not burn trash or scrap wood in your backyard.

> Take special precautions if there is a wildfire near your community.

3 THE INDOOR AIR WE BREATHE

Fresh air keeps the doctor poor.

Danish proverb

YOU SHOULD BE able to think of your home as a sanctuary, a place where you are safe from the tumult and troubles of the outside world. From this perspective, it's disturbing to learn that indoor air pollution poses serious threats to our health. When most people think about poor air quality, they think about smog and other types of outdoor air pollution. Yet the U.S. Environmental Protection Agency ranks indoor air pollution as one of the top five environmental threats to health. Indoor air is a crucial influence on your health because you spend roughly 87% of your time inside buildings, with about 6% of your time in vehicles and 7% outdoors.

Indoor air in a typical home may contain hundreds of toxic substances, including radon, a radioactive gas; lead; by-products of burning tobacco, oil, gas, and wood; volatile organic compounds; and biological contaminants such as mold and dust mites. As well, pollutants from outdoor air penetrate residential buildings of all types—detached homes, apartments, condominiums, and townhouses. Pollutants from traffic and industry are more likely to be present at health-threatening levels in indoor air in low-income neighborhoods.

Millions of people suffer from respiratory illnesses either caused by or exacerbated by air pollution. Asthma is a respiratory disorder that causes wheezing, coughing, difficulty breathing, and tightness in the chest. It can be triggered by either outdoor or indoor air pollution, and is one of the leading causes of school and workplace absence. Rates of asthma have skyrocketed in some industrialized nations. Asthma affects more than 20 million Americans, including more than 6 million children. In 2000, asthma caused 14 million missed school days, 3 million lost workdays, 2 million emergency room visits, and half a million hospitalizations in the U.S., at a cost of billions of dollars. Over 2.7 million Canadians and more than 2 million Australians suffer from asthma. From 1978 to 1999, the percentage of Canadian children with asthma quadrupled to its current level of more than 12%. In Canada, asthma causes hundreds of deaths each year and is the leading cause of emergency room visits, the leading reason for absence from school, and the third leading reason for absence from work. An Australian study estimated that poor indoor air quality costs that nation $12 billion annually.

> **An airtight energy-conserving house can have worse air quality than a "leaky" one because pollutants from indoor activities, building materials, and consumer products become trapped inside**

Allergies are the body's response to a number of triggers called allergens. Many types of indoor air pollution are potent allergens. Experts estimate that one person in ten is allergic to mold, with allergic responses ranging from itchy eyes, runny nose, and sneezing to asthma. Although generally mild, allergic reactions can be severe enough to cause death. Illnesses such as sick building syndrome (symptoms of acute discomfort experienced by building occupants) and multiple chemical sensitivity syndrome (unusually severe reactions to low levels of chemical exposure) are also linked to indoor air quality problems.

In recent decades, efforts to solve one environmental problem have inadvertently led to another. Conservation measures initiated in the 1970s to make buildings more energy efficient have reduced ventilation dramatically. Today an airtight energy-conserving house can have worse air quality than a "leaky" one because pollutants from indoor activities, building materials, and consumer products become trapped inside.

Major Indoor Air Pollutants

We are all vulnerable to the adverse effects of indoor air pollution, which involves many compounds and contaminants, including tobacco smoke, radon, volatile organic compounds, combustion by-products, biological contaminants, and asbestos.

Three basic strategies can improve indoor air quality:

1. Reducing pollutants at the source (preventing pollution in the first place).

2. Increasing ventilation (diluting and removing pollutants by exchanging fresh air for stale air).

3. Installing machines that filter air (not to be confused with plug-in air fresheners or sprays, which actually worsen indoor air quality by releasing noxious chemicals).

Tobacco Smoke

There are more than 4,000 toxic substances in tobacco smoke, including hydrogen cyanide, arsenic, benzene, formaldehyde, cadmium, vinyl chloride, 4-aminobiphenyl, acrylonitrile, benzo[a]pyrene, and 1,3-butadiene. Smoking and exposure to secondhand smoke remain major public health issues throughout the world, despite declining smoking rates in industrialized countries. Smoking is one of the primary causes of cancer, heart disease, and respiratory ailments. It causes millions of deaths globally every year. Smoking also exacerbates the risks posed by other environmental hazards. For example, the risks of lung cancer caused by exposure to radon or asbestos increase at a much higher rate for smokers.

Secondhand smoke (also called environmental tobacco smoke) causes cancer, heart disease, and respiratory illness. Exposure to the secondhand smoke from just one cigarette per day accelerates the progression of atherosclerosis (the hardening and narrowing of the arteries). Thousands of nonsmoking Canadians, Americans, and Australians die annually because of lung cancer and heart disease caused by exposure to secondhand smoke. Living with a smoker increases your risk of lung cancer by up to 30% and your risk of heart disease by up to 35%.

Despite a decline in smoking rates, one in two adults and one in three children are still exposed to secondhand smoke. Children exposed to tobacco smoke are more likely to suffer from lung problems, ear infections, and asthma. In the U.S., experts estimate that exposure to secondhand smoke causes children to suffer up to 1 million asthma attacks, between 150,000 and 300,000 lower respiratory tract infections (e.g., bronchitis, pneumonia), and 7,500 to 15,000 hospitalizations linked to these afflictions every year. Exposure to secondhand smoke is also likely to play a role in sudden infant death syndrome (SIDS).

WHAT YOU CAN DO

> Do not smoke or allow smoking in your home or vehicle.

> Support businesses—restaurants, bars, hotels—that are completely smoke-free. Separate no-smoking sections and open windows will not adequately protect you and your family from the health hazards posed by tobacco smoke.

> Ask people not to smoke around you and your family. This is particularly important for the health of young children.

> Insist that your employer provide a smoke-free workplace. This is a legal requirement in most jurisdictions.

> Support laws that restrict smoking in public places, ban advertising of tobacco products, and prohibit the sale of tobacco products to children and youths. The American Cancer Society and the International Union Against Cancer provide an outstanding series of strategic guides for tobacco control advocacy at http://strategyguides.globalink.org.

> Donate to advocacy groups that promote smoking reduction strategies: Physicians for a Smoke-free Canada (www.smoke-free.ca), Canadian Council for Tobacco Control (www.cctc.ca), American Cancer Society (www.cancer.org), Action on Smoking and Health (www.ash.org), Canadian Cancer Society (www.cancer.ca), and Cancer Council Australia (www.cancer.org.au).

> Help family, friends, colleagues, and other people who are trying to quit smoking. Various organizations offer advice on this topic, including the American Lung Association (www.lungusa.org), the Australian Lung Foundation (www.lungfoundation.com.au), and the Canadian Lung Association (www.lung.ca).

Radon

Radon is a naturally occurring gas that comes from the decay of uranium and other radioactive elements distributed throughout soil and rocks in varying concentrations. Certain geographic regions face higher radon risks than others, but any building anywhere may have elevated radon levels. Radon seeps into buildings through cracks and other weaknesses in foundations and floors. While radon may also be present in drinking water and outdoor air, exposure occurs most commonly through indoor air. It surprises many people to learn that radon is the second most important cause of lung cancer after smoking and the number one cause of lung cancer among nonsmokers. Annually, radon kills roughly twenty-one thousand people in the U.S., twenty thousand people in Europe, and two thousand people in Canada. Radon levels in Australia are much lower than in Europe and North America.

Radon reduction systems can lower radon levels in your home by up to 99%

Nearly one out of every fifteen homes in the U.S. is estimated to have an elevated radon level. The good news is that it is not expensive to measure radon concentrations in your home and take steps to avoid exposure. Testing for radon levels generally costs less than $50. Radon reduction systems can lower radon levels in your home by up to 99%. The cost of fixing a home generally ranges from $800 to $2,500 (with an average cost of about $1,200). Costs will vary depending on the size and design of your home and which radon reduction methods are needed. Hundreds of thousands of people have successfully reduced radon levels in their homes. Construction techniques for new buildings can easily incorporate radon reduction features at minimal cost.

WHAT YOU CAN DO

> Have your home tested for radon if you live in a house or on the ground floor in an apartment or condominium building. In the U.S., you can purchase a home testing kit from the National Safety Council or have testing done by a certified professional. Call 1-800-SOS-RADON (767-7236). Canadians can buy radon testing kits over the Internet.

> If tests indicate that your radon level exceeds 4 picoCuries per liter (150 bequerels per cubic meter), then it is essential to fix your home. Otherwise you and your family face substantially higher risks of developing lung cancer.

> The most effective way to reduce radon levels in buildings is depressurization, which involves installing vent pipes to redirect radon-containing air outside the building. Active ventilation (using fans or air conditioning) is moderately effective. Passive ventilation (opening doors and windows) and sealing cracks in floors and walls is ineffective. Retest radon levels after installation to make sure the problem is solved.

> Learn more about radon. In the U.S., extensive information is available through the Environmental Protection Agency. See "A Citizen's Guide to Radon," "Home Buyer's and Seller's Guide to Radon," and "Consumer's Guide to Radon Reduction," all available at www.epa.gov/radon. In Canada, see "Radon: A Guide for Canadian Homeowners" at www.healthcanada.gc.ca/radon.

Volatile Organic Compounds

Volatile organic compounds (VOCs) are gases emitted by various products, including paints, varnishes, paint strippers, wood preservatives, mothballs, cleaning supplies, fabric softeners, dryer sheets, hair spray, dry-cleaned clothing, air fresheners, windshield washer fluid, liquid fuels, building materials, furnishings, office equipment, glues and adhesives, permanent markers, and photographic solutions. VOC levels are generally higher indoors than outdoors, and can be up to a thousand times higher than normal during activities such as paint stripping.

VOC levels are generally higher indoors than outdoors, and can be up to a thousand times higher than normal during activities such as paint stripping

Exposure to VOCs can cause immediate health effects, including eye, nose, skin, and throat irritation; headaches; loss of coordination and confusion; nausea and vomiting; and difficulty breathing. Repeated exposure to VOCs can cause serious long-term effects such as cancer, and damage to the liver, kidneys, and central nervous system, harming both physical and mental health (see page 61). VOCs are particularly problematic for people suffering from chemical sensitivities. Many factors will determine if exposure to VOCs makes you sick, including the concentration and amount of the chemical; your age, gender, weight, and general health status; the route of exposure (by inhalation or direct contact with your skin); whether one or multiple chemicals are involved; and the duration of the exposure (longer exposures cause greater risk).

WHAT YOU CAN DO

> Avoid purchasing products that contain VOCs. In many cases, safer substitutes exist. Water-based paint releases far fewer VOCs than oil-based paint. Buy no-VOC or low-VOC products. They may be marginally more expensive, but your health is worth the additional cost. Look for paints, stains, adhesives, cleaners, building materials, furnishings, and other products certified by GreenGuard, Green Seal, GreenSpec, or another respected certification organization.

> When using products that emit even low amounts of VOCs, follow directions on the label, increase the supply of fresh air, and meet or exceed any label precautions. Whenever possible, it is better to use such products outside where there is maximum air circulation. If you must work indoors, maximize ventilation using fans, and open doors or windows and take plenty of breaks. Vent fumes out the window rather than to the rest of the house. Consider using a respirator approved by NIOSH (the National Institute for Occupational Safety and Health), with activated carbon filter cartridges to absorb the VOCs. Keep children out of the affected area.

> Make an extra effort to avoid six of the most hazardous VOCs: benzene, formaldehyde, toluene, methylene chloride, paradichlorobenzene, and perchloroethylene.

  · The main indoor sources of benzene are tobacco smoke, stored fuels, and paint supplies.

  · Formaldehyde is found commonly in pressed wood products (e.g., plywood, particle board, medium-density fiber-board, and oriented strand board). Use solid wood products instead of these when possible. If buying pressed wood products, choose those certified by the Forest Stewardship Council to reduce formaldehyde exposure. If you have pressed wood products in your home, coat or seal them with a no- or low-VOC surface finish.

  · Toluene is used in household aerosols, nail polish, paints and paint thinners, lacquers, rust inhibitors, adhesives, and solvent-based cleaning agents. It is also found in tobacco smoke and vehicle emissions.

  · Methylene chloride is often found in paint strippers, adhesive removers, and aerosol spray paints. Minimize your use of these products and look for brands that do not list methylene chloride among their ingredients.

- Paradichlorobenzene is mainly used to kill moths. Instead of bringing mothballs into your home, try one of the safer cedar products that are available. Paradichlorobenzene is also used in puck form and sprays for public washrooms and diaper pails. Ask management of facilities not to use these products, and do not use them yourself.

- Find a dry cleaner that does not use perchloroethylene. Otherwise, allow dry-cleaning to air out for a week in a garage, outbuilding, or part of your home that is not regularly occupied.

> Buy limited quantities of products containing VOCs, so that you will not need to store these products at your home.

> Dispose of unwanted or unused products safely and immediately, as gases may leak from closed containers. In most communities, local governments and recycling centers offer occasional collection days for toxic household products. If storage is necessary, use a well-ventilated area that is inaccessible to young children and pets.

> Avoid so-called air fresheners and deodorizers, especially the plug-in variety, as the chemicals released by these products often include phthalates (see Chapter 6) and may react with other air pollutants in the home to create formaldehyde. Identify and remove the sources of any undesirable odors and use baking soda and vinegar to keep your home smelling fresh.

> Replace carpets (which emit VOCs) with wood, ceramic tile, natural linoleum, bamboo, or other sustainable materials. Use small area rugs that can be thoroughly cleaned. Avoid flooring, window blinds, or wall coverings made with polyvinyl chloride, which is linked to decreased lung function.

> Place photocopiers, printers, photography development equipment, and similar items in rooms that are vented to the outside or have special ventilation systems.

> Air out newly built, newly renovated, or newly furnished areas with fresh, clean outdoor air for a minimum of one week or until the new odors dissipate. This is particularly important for mobile homes and other portable buildings.

> Use fragrance-free cleaners and polishes that you rub on rather than spray. Cleaning sprays cause increased asthma symptoms. Avoid cleaners that have warnings on the label such as Danger, Flammable, or Caution.

Combustion Products

Gas and oil furnaces, woodstoves, fireplaces, unvented gas and kerosene space heaters, and gas kitchen stoves can all release air pollutants, including carbon monoxide, nitrogen dioxide, and particulate matter. Combustion gases and small particles also come from chimneys and flues that are improperly installed or maintained. The adverse health effects of these pollutants are well known. Pollutants from fireplaces and woodstoves with no dedicated outdoor air supply can back-draft from chimneys into your home, particularly in airtight buildings. Hundreds of people die every year from carbon monoxide poisoning that occurs when gas appliances are not working properly or are being used incorrectly. According to the *Journal of the American Medical Association,* carbon monoxide is one of the leading causes of accidental poisoning deaths in the U.S. Idling vehicles in garages, parkades, or other enclosed spaces also pose a serious threat of carbon monoxide poisoning.

Hundreds of people die every year from carbon monoxide poisoning that occurs when gas appliances are not working properly or are being used incorrectly

Wood smoke from stoves, fireplaces, and boilers deserves special attention because so many people mistakenly regard it as harmless. With rising energy prices you may be tempted to switch to good old-fashioned wood. Unfortunately, any savings on fuel costs are likely to be exceeded by extra health costs. An Australian study estimated that the annual costs of illness and death caused by the operation of a single woodstove

>> MENTAL HEALTH AND THE ENVIRONMENT

THE IMPACTS OF environmental hazards on mental health are often overlooked. Chemicals can have major effects on brain function, as demonstrated by alcohol, marijuana, and other drugs. Involuntary exposure to toxic substances can also upset the complex chemistry involved in proper brain function. Among the adverse mental health effects associated with exposure to toxic chemicals are diminished intellectual capacity, emotional and behavioral dysfunction, depression, memory problems, sleep disturbance, impaired concentration, and various other difficulties.

A 2006 article in *The Lancet* warned that we are harming millions of children across the world by exposing them to industrial chemicals. It is well established that five substances—lead, mercury, arsenic, PCBs, and toluene—cause neurological disorders and brain dysfunction in babies and young children. Hundreds of other industrial chemicals—including pesticides, solvents, and heavy metals—are suspected of being developmental neurotoxins, but the evidence is not yet conclusive. The neurodevelopmental disorders and deficits caused by industrial chemicals include attention deficit hyperactivity disorder, mental retardation, cerebral palsy, autism spectrum disorders, and decreased cognition, memory, and intelligence. Researchers have linked childhood lead exposure to criminal behavior later in life, finding a strong association between the blood lead levels of preschoolers and the rates of serious crimes such as murder, rape, and aggravated assault two decades later—when the preschoolers have grown up. Similarly, teenage boys with elevated lead levels have been found to engage in bullying, vandalism, arson, shoplifting, and other socially undesirable behavior more often than boys with normal lead levels. Because neurodevelopmental damage is generally irreversible, preventing exposure is the only responsible option.

approached $2,000. In parts of the U.S., Canada, and Australia, wood-stoves and fireplaces are the largest residential source of particulate matter. Even the best new models generate significantly more particle pollution than comparable oil or gas heaters. In addition to particulate matter, wood smoke emissions may contain carbon monoxide, nitrogen dioxide, sulfur dioxide, hydrochloric acid, and known or suspected carcinogens, such as polycyclic aromatic hydrocarbons, formaldehyde, and dioxin. Exposure to wood smoke can cause respiratory problems, exacerbate asthma, and decrease your body's ability to resist disease.

WHAT YOU CAN DO

> Never idle your vehicle in a garage or other enclosed space. Keep doors between the house and attached garages closed.

> Choose appliances that vent their fumes to the outside and have them properly installed. Keep your fuel-burning appliances properly maintained and have them inspected by a professional annually. Follow operating and maintenance instructions for all fuel-burning devices.

> Replace old woodstoves with new clean-burning high-efficiency models (or an ultraefficient pellet stove) and burn only dry, well-aged wood. Always open flues on fireplaces. Make sure doors on woodstoves fit tightly. Use only newspaper and small kindling to start your fire. Small pieces of wood burn hotter, producing less smoke. Never burn painted or treated wood, garbage, colored paper, or pressed wood products like plywood. These items release harmful chemicals and excess smoke as they burn. Visible smoke from your chimney is a sign of incomplete combustion.

> Never use the burners or oven of a gas stove to heat your home, even for a short time. Vent gas stoves to the outside by using a range hood with an exhaust fan. When you buy a new stove, look for one with an electric ignition instead of a pilot light that is always burning.

> Never use a charcoal grill or gas barbecue indoors.

> Do not sleep in a room with an unvented gas or kerosene space heater. Always keep a window slightly open when using these products.

> Never use any gasoline-powered engines (e.g., mowers, weed trimmers, snowblowers, chain saws, small engines, or generators) in enclosed spaces. Store these items in a location separate from your home.

> Use carbon monoxide detectors for backup only, as they are no substitute for maintaining and using fuel-burning appliances properly. According to the U.S. Environmental Protection Agency, their performance is not as reliable as smoke detectors. If you buy a carbon monoxide detector, make sure it is independently certified (e.g., by Underwriters Laboratories) and carefully follow the manufacturer's instructions for placement, use, and maintenance.

Biological Contaminants

Biological contaminants include bacteria, viruses, molds, mildew, dust mites, cockroaches, and pollen, as well as animal dander (minute pieces of skin, hair, or feathers), saliva, and droppings—anything living or once part of a living organism. Some biological contaminants can trigger asthma and allergic reactions. For example, urine from rats and mice is a potent allergen that can become airborne when it dries. Spores from molds and mildews growing in homes and on building materials can release disease-causing toxins. Moisture problems in as many as one in three homes in North America and Europe increase the likelihood of mold growth. Although people can be exposed to mold through food and direct contact, most exposures result from breathing contaminated indoor air.

Spores from molds and mildews growing in homes and on building materials can release disease-causing toxins

Symptoms caused by biological contaminants include sneezing, watery eyes, coughing, shortness of breath, dizziness, lethargy, fever, and digestive disturbances. Health problems include some potentially serious lung infections. For example, contact with airborne particles from mouse droppings can cause hantavirus infection, a flu-like illness. If heating and cooling systems are not properly maintained, they can become breeding grounds for mold, mildew, and other biological contaminants and can distribute these health hazards throughout buildings. Children, the elderly, and people with respiratory problems and allergies are particularly vulnerable to biological contaminants in indoor air.

WHAT YOU CAN DO

> Keep your home clean. Remove shoes at the door. Use a vacuum with a HEPA (high efficiency particulate air) filter to regularly clean flooring, furniture, and window coverings.

> Control the relative humidity level in your home, keeping it in the range of 30% to 50%.

> Install and use exhaust fans vented to the outdoors in bathrooms and kitchens.

> Ventilate attics and crawl spaces to prevent excessive moisture levels.

> If you use a humidifier, follow the instructions and replace water regularly.

> Vent clothes dryers to the outside.

> Wash bedding in hot water weekly to kill dust mites. Use dust-proof covers on pillows and mattresses. Freezing pillows and stuffed toys will kill mites but will not remove existing allergenic particles.

> Address mold problems by:

　· Immediately repairing areas where water has leaked and replacing all damaged materials.

　· Replacing carpets with tiles, wood, or other forms of flooring.

　· Regularly cleaning bathroom areas where mold may develop, such as grout, caulking, and shower curtains.

- Regularly inspecting basements and garages for moisture.

- Watching for mold in old books and newspapers, firewood, and drip pans for fridges and freezers, and then cleaning or discarding if necessary.

- Increasing air movement in your home.

Asbestos

Asbestos was once considered a "miracle" mineral for its ability to withstand heat. It was used in thousands of products, including fireproofing and insulating material in buildings and consumer products, wallboard, flooring, cement, automobiles, clothing, home appliances, and children's toys. As it turned out, asbestos can have devastating effects on health, and its widespread use was one of the greatest public health disasters of the twentieth century. The World Health Organization estimates that asbestos exposure kills more than ninety thousand people annually, including thousands of North Americans, by causing mesothelioma, lung cancer, and asbestosis. These diseases may take twenty to forty years to develop following exposure to asbestos fibers (see page 66).

The World Health Organization estimates that asbestos exposure kills more than ninety thousand people annually

While often thought of as primarily an occupational hazard, asbestos can also harm the families of workers in asbestos industries, people living near asbestos mines or manufacturing facilities, and anyone exposed to asbestos at home, school, or work. For example, women living in asbestos mining communities in Quebec suffer from cancer at seven times the normal rate. Critical factors in determining your risk are the concentration of fibers in the air and the length of exposure. In addition to the enormous health costs and the incalculable human suffering, the legal costs of the asbestos disaster are astronomical. In the U.S., more than six hundred thousand people have been involved in lawsuits stemming from their exposure to asbestos, at a cost of more than US$50 billion. Up to 3 million people may eventually sue, with estimated costs as high as US$265 billion.

ASBESTOS: A PREVENTABLE TRAGEDY ≪

Conclusive evidence that all forms of asbestos are carcinogenic has led most industrialized nations to follow the World Health Organization's advice and ban these hazardous substances. Most asbestos use in the world today is in developing nations. To its shame, Canada is one of the world's largest asbestos exporters, with over 95% of Canadian asbestos going to developing nations. Indefensibly, Canada joined forces with Zimbabwe, Iran, and Kazakhstan to block international efforts to add asbestos to the list of hazardous materials regulated by the Rotterdam Convention. This means there is now no requirement for Canada and other asbestos-exporting nations to follow a prior informed consent procedure that alerts importing nations to the threats posed by a substance known for causing devastating health impacts in the industrialized world during the twentieth century. The epidemic of death and disease caused by asbestos should be prevented rather than repeated in developing nations in the twenty-first century.

Many building products and types of insulation used in the past contain asbestos: blankets or tape for insulating boilers, steam pipes, and furnace ducts; door gaskets in furnaces and woodstoves; soundproofing or decorative materials sprayed on walls or ceilings; automobile brake pads; and patching and joint compounds for walls, ceilings, and textured paints. When asbestos-containing products or materials are worn down, sanded, scraped, or otherwise disturbed, they may release asbestos fibers. The main sources of asbestos in a home are asbestos-containing insulation, ceiling tiles, and floor tiles that are damaged or deteriorating.

WHAT YOU CAN DO

> If your home was built before 1970 and you suspect that it contains asbestos materials, seek professional advice before beginning any major renovations. Asbestos removal businesses can be located using the Yellow Pages or the Internet.

> Generally, material in good condition will not release asbestos fibers. Danger only arises when asbestos materials decay or are disturbed and release fibers that can be inhaled. Often the best thing is to simply leave asbestos material that is in good condition alone. Check it regularly (without touching it) to watch for signs of wear and tear or damage such as abrasions or water damage.

> Discard damaged or worn products that may contain asbestos, such as older stovetop pads, ironing board covers, and woodstove door gaskets. Check with local health and environmental officials to find out proper handling and disposal procedures.

> Never saw, sand, scrape, or drill holes in asbestos materials.

> Do not dust, sweep, or vacuum debris that may contain asbestos, as these activities increase the risk of inhalation. Use a wet mop, or call an asbestos removal professional. Ordinary dust masks provide no protection against asbestos because the fibers are so small.

Air Cleaners

Using machines to clean your air falls a distant third behind the first and second best ways to ensure you breathe safe indoor air—preventing pollution at the source and keeping your home adequately ventilated. Some air cleaners are effective at removing particles from the air but few are good at removing gases such as VOCs, nitrogen oxides, or carbon monoxide. There are four main types of air cleaners:

- Mechanical filters can be installed on your furnace, air conditioner, or as part of your ventilation system. There are also stand-alone devices designed to capture particles from the air in room-sized areas. HEPA filters are the best available technology and must be replaced according to the manufacturer's instructions to be effective. Activated carbon filters will trap VOCs, but in order to be effective, a large quantity of filter medium is needed, and this requires frequent replacement.

- Electronic air cleaners use an electrical field to trap particles. They can be a part of the ventilation system or a stand-alone device. Electronic air cleaners do not remove gases or odors and produce health-harming ozone as a by-product.

- Ion generators are portable units that use static charges to trap particles. Most ion generators do not remove gases or odors, and they are relatively ineffective in removing large particles such as pollen and house dust. Ion generators produce health-harming ozone as a by-product.

- Hybrid models of air cleaners incorporate two or more of the filtering systems mentioned above.

The value of any air cleaner depends on its efficiency and its suitability for removing a particular type of pollutant. Proper installation and regular maintenance are required, along with the recognition of possible drawbacks: inadequate pollutant removal, masking of pollution rather than removal, ozone production, and unacceptable noise levels.

A superior alternative to air cleaners may be houseplants. Certain types of plants improve indoor air quality by absorbing pollutants such as VOCS and small particles. A recent study estimated that fifteen to twenty houseplants could purify the air of a typical 150-square-meter (1,600-square-foot) house. It is worth noting that some plants are toxic if ingested and should be kept away from young children and pets. As well, houseplants can be a trigger for asthma and allergies, and may not be appropriate for people with these conditions. The following are reputed to be the most effective at cleaning indoor air:

- money tree (*Pachira aquatica*)
- spider plant (*Chlorophytum comosum*)
- English ivy (*Hedera helix*)
- bamboo palm (*Chamaedorea sefritzii*)
- weeping fig (*Ficus benjamina*)
- rubber plant (*Ficus elastica*)
- devil's ivy (*Scindapsus aureus*)
- African daisy (*Gerbera jamesonii*)
- snake plant (*Sansevieria trifasciata*)
- philodendrons, all kinds (*Philodendron*)
- dracaenas, all kinds (*Dracaena*)
- Chinese evergreen, all kinds (*Aglaonema*)

Advice for Parents

Children are especially vulnerable to many indoor air pollutants. Rates of childhood asthma have skyrocketed in recent years, especially in poor urban neighborhoods. Protect your children by taking these steps:

> Never let anyone smoke near your children.

> Ideally, undertake renovation and painting projects before a child is even conceived, airing out the affected areas well. The developing fetus is extremely sensitive to toxic substances found in common household items, including paint, carpet, and furniture.

> Address contamination problems related to insects, mold, and rodents.

> Replace wall-to-wall carpeting and heavy curtains or window coverings that need to be dry-cleaned, as these are all reservoirs for dust and pollutants.

> Keep children away from areas where painting, gluing, varnishing, and other activities produce high levels of VOCs.

> Wash stuffed toys in hot water regularly and dry them completely to minimize exposure to dust mites, which can trigger asthma attacks.

Wrap-up

Individuals can protect themselves from some hazards associated with indoor air quality, but government has an important role to play as well. Governments often turn a blind eye to many indoor air issues. For example, in the aftermath of Hurricane Katrina, thousands of Americans were exposed to unhealthy levels of formaldehyde while housed temporarily in mobile homes. More recently, alarm bells rang about toxic substances in drywall imported from China. When governments do address indoor air quality, they often rely on weak, unenforceable guidelines instead of effective, legally binding rules. Despite the well-established dangers of radon in the U.S. and Canada, only a small proportion of homeowners have tested their homes or taken steps to address the problem. Stronger policies are needed. In areas where radon occurs at dangerous levels, building codes should require radon protection measures in all new construction. Mandatory disclosure of radon levels should be required when homes are sold. Financial support for testing should be available in low-income areas, and, if necessary, public buildings such as schools, daycare facilities, and hospitals should be renovated to reduce radon levels.

In cases where indoor air policies have been introduced and enforced, progress has been made. When Helena, Montana, banned smoking in public places for six months in 2002, there was a 40% decline in hospital admissions for heart attacks—a decline that was not found in any other Montana community. New standards for wood-burning stoves are much more protective of human health and the environment than their predecessors.

While the emphasis in this chapter is on indoor air quality in your home, the same problems exist and the same solutions apply in schools, hospitals, workplaces, and commercial buildings. According to the U.S. Environmental Protection Agency, one in two schools suffers from indoor air quality problems, mainly related to molds and VOCs. Poor indoor air quality may be encountered in almost any setting. Figure skaters and hockey players often suffer from respiratory problems because of poor air quality in indoor ice arenas. Indoor swimming pools may be linked to asthma because of gases formed by chlorine reactions, although more research is needed and swimming is generally a healthy activity. Less surprisingly, research proves that poor air quality jeopardizes health at indoor motor shows such as monster truck competitions. Wherever you spend time, be alert to potential hazards and take steps to protect your health.

Breathe Clean Indoor Air

> Make your home a no-smoking zone.

> Determine whether you face any risks from radon or asbestos and take remedial action if required.

> Keep gas-, oil-, and wood-burning stoves, heaters, and appliances in good condition.

> Buy low- or no-VOC products.

> Remove your shoes at the door to avoid tracking contaminants into your home, clean your home regularly, and use a vacuum with a HEPA (high efficiency particulate air) filter on flooring, window coverings, and furniture.

> Ensure that ventilation is adequate.

> Keep the relative humidity in your home between 30% and 50%.

4 THE FOOD WE EAT

Eat food, not too much, mostly plants.

Michael Pollan, author of *An Omnivore's Dilemma* and *In Defense of Food*

FOOD IS THE renewable energy that powers us and provides all the nutrients we need to be healthy—carbohydrates, proteins, vitamins, essential fatty acids, trace elements, and roughage (the indigestible components of plants). Millions of cells in our bodies die daily and must be replaced. Our remarkable digestive system employs everything from hydrochloric acid to helpful kinds of bacteria, converting food into the smaller molecules that our bodies rely upon to form bones, blood, and flesh. Like goats, rats, and cockroaches, we eat a wide range of foods and our omnivorous appetite is a major factor in our evolutionary success, enabling us to live in many different ecosystems.

Today more than ever before, processing and packaging obscure the fact that virtually every type of food providing us with nutritional value comes from other living things. Food comes from the Earth, not a factory, laboratory, or supermarket. We are what we eat. The plants and animals that make up our diet have inhaled, ingested, and absorbed whatever is in the air, water, and soil. By contaminating the environment with toxic substances, we set off a chain reaction that ultimately leads back to our own bodies. Our coal-fired power plants spew mercury into the air.

The mercury rains down into oceans, lakes, and rivers, moves through aquatic food chains into fish, and we eat the fish, jeopardizing our health and, more acutely, the health of our infants and children. The flame retardants we add to carpets and furniture eventually enter the environment and accumulate in the fatty tissue of animals, making their way back to us in beef, pork, dairy products, and eggs. Hormones, antibiotics, and even arsenic take a more direct path to us when we feed them to livestock that we subsequently consume. What goes around, comes around.

Today's diets are making us sick, and in some cases the food we eat is killing us. Through food we are exposed to harmful bacteria and viruses, heavy metals, persistent organic pollutants such as dioxins, pesticides, antibiotics, and growth hormones. In 2008, a *Listeria* outbreak caused by contaminated cold cuts led to twenty deaths in Canada. In 2009, a *Salmonella* outbreak related to peanuts caused more than 640 confirmed illnesses in the U.S. and was linked to at least ten deaths. Tens of millions of Americans, Canadians, and Australians become ill and thousands die from foodborne illnesses every year.

Reducing our exposure to environmental hazards in food is a straightforward process. We need to identify the main sources of contaminants and unhealthy additives in order to avoid the foods that make us sick. But before we do this by taking a virtual trip around the grocery store, stopping at the meat and dairy department, the fish counter, the fresh produce section, and the processed food aisles, we need to consider another essential step. First and foremost, we need to stop eating more food than our bodies require.

The Perils of Overeating

In the industrialized nations, for the first time in human history, more people suffer poor health because of overconsumption than starvation or malnutrition. It's not just the people who set world records in eating contests by stuffing themselves in ten minutes on sixty-eight hot dogs (bun included), four kilograms of meatballs, or 231 chicken and vegetable gyozas. Globally, more than 1 billion people are now overweight, and rates of obesity are soaring among adults and children alike. In fact, over the past twenty-five years the proportion of obese children has doubled in Canada and tripled in the U.S. and Australia.

People, including children, are consuming unprecedented quantities of junk food, fast food, and processed food, resulting in diets where a disproportionate number of calories come from high-fat and high-sugar foods. Between 1977 and 2002, the average American child's consumption of candy doubled, while the consumption of salty snacks tripled and the consumption of pizza quadrupled. At the same time, children's intake of vegetables declined and soft drinks replaced milk as the dominant beverage for children and teenagers. Overall, less than one in ten Americans eats a healthy diet. Meanwhile, people are sitting in front of televisions and computers for an increasing proportion of their time. The epidemic of obesity that has resulted is far more damaging to human health than exposure to environmental hazards through diet.

Obesity is costing society hundreds of billions of dollars annually, a gargantuan sum that rivals the costs of smoking

As noted in Chapter 1, for the first time in more than a century, children face shorter life expectancies than their parents. The main culprit is diabetes, which is directly linked to obesity, which in turn is often connected to overeating. Diabetes increases the risk of heart disease, stroke, blindness, kidney failure, and limb loss. Obesity is linked to an array of medical problems, including increased risk of heart attack and stroke, hypertension, gall bladder disease, osteoarthritis of the knee, and endometrial cancer. Estimates of obesity-related deaths in the U.S. range from 112,000 to 400,000 per year. Obesity is costing society hundreds of billions of dollars annually, a gargantuan sum that rivals the costs of smoking. According to the World Health Organization, "without societal changes, a substantial and steadily rising proportion of adults will succumb to the medical complications of obesity; indeed, the medical burden of obesity already threatens to overwhelm health services... obesity should be regarded as today's principal neglected public health problem."

WHAT YOU CAN DO

> Eat smaller meals, perhaps consuming one helping instead of two. The long-lived Japanese residents of Okinawa, who reach the ripe old age of one hundred more often than anyone else in the world, have a cultural practice called *hara hachi bu*, which means stop eating when you are 80% full.

> Strive to eat healthy, wholesome foods, with a focus on fruits and vegetables.

> Eat a balanced and nutritious breakfast to set a good tone for the day.

> Cut back on junk food, fast food, and processed food, including soft drinks.

The Meat and Dairy Department

Individual Americans, Canadians, and Australians are a carnivorous bunch, consuming about 100 kilograms (220 pounds) of meat a year. This works out to 275 grams (9 ounces) a day (equal to three big burger patties), twice the global average and three times more than the amount recommended by the World Cancer Research Fund. Meat is a major source of exposure to persistent organic pollutants, foodborne pathogens, heavy metals, antibiotics, and hormones. High levels of meat consumption increase the risk of a Pandora's box of chronic health problems, including heart disease, stroke, cancer, and gallbladder disease. In particular, long-term consumption of red meat and processed meat increases the risk of esophageal, liver, and colorectal cancer. Recent studies investigating the health of American women revealed a strong association between higher red meat consumption and elevated risk of breast cancer. There are also continuing concerns about so-called bird flu, swine flu, and mad cow disease (bovine spongiform encephalopathy or BSE), infectious diseases linked to industrialized meat production.

Persistent Organic Pollutants

Persistent organic pollutants (POPs) can build up in our bodies over a lifetime, causing adverse health effects. To make matters worse, POPs can be passed on to our children, who may suffer health impacts later in their lives as a result. Dioxins are the most notorious POPs. One specific type of dioxin, 2,3,7,8-TCDD, appears to be the most potent carcinogen discovered, meaning it can cause cancer at extraordinarily low levels of exposure. Dioxins are also linked to cardiovascular disease, diabetes, learning disorders, immune system disorders, and damage to the reproductive system. The average person's body contains tiny amounts of dioxins, yet these low levels may be sufficient to cause adverse health effects. The World Health Organization has repeatedly lowered its estimate of the safe level of dioxin exposure for humans. While their use is banned, dioxins continue to be created as a by-product of industrial processes, the burning of plastics, and natural events such as volcanic eruptions and forest fires. In the U.S., backyard burning is the number one source of dioxins.

> Governments estimate that meat, dairy, poultry, and fish products contribute over 90% of our exposure to dioxins

Tests conducted by the Canadian Food Inspection Agency found dioxins in almost all samples of beef fat and raw milk tested, and in most samples of chicken fat, mutton fat, and pork fat. Under Canadian law, it is illegal to sell these contaminated products, but the government turns a blind eye to its own rules. It is likely that similar American and Australian foods also contain dioxins. Governments estimate that meat, dairy, poultry, and fish products contribute over 90% of our exposure to dioxins. There are seventy-five forms of chlorinated dioxins, but only a minority are commonly monitored and regulated. Dioxins that contaminate common herbicides are not among them, although one is known to be as potent as 2,3,7,8-TCDD in suppressing the immune system—an important step in the development of cancers and other illnesses.

Foodborne Pathogens

Meat consumption also poses a threat of immediate illness through microbial contamination. Indeed, the majority of foodborne illnesses can be traced to items of animal origin—meat, poultry, fish, dairy products, and eggs (see page 80). Young children, elderly people, pregnant women, and individuals with compromised immune systems are particularly vulnerable. Five pathogens account for 90% of food-related deaths and the majority of foodborne illnesses in the U.S. and Canada: *Salmonella, Listeria, Toxoplasma, Campylobacter,* and *E. coli.*

Undercooked hamburger meat and poorly washed lettuce are two common sources of *E. coli* O157:H7. Consumption of food contaminated with this bacteria can lead to serious and life-threatening illnesses. Symptoms include severe abdominal pain and bloody diarrhea. Some people may have seizures or strokes and some may need blood transfusions and kidney dialysis. Others may live with permanent kidney damage.

More than 80% of chickens harbor *Campylobacter,* while another 15% harbor *Salmonella. Campylobacter* may cause diarrhea, abdominal pain, fever, nausea, muscle pain, and headache. In rare cases, it may also lead to meningitis, arthritis, and Guillain-Barré syndrome, a severe neurological disorder. Salmonellosis may cause short-term symptoms such as high fever, severe headache, vomiting, nausea, abdominal pain, and diarrhea. Long-term complications may include severe arthritis.

Listeria is detected in the majority of ground beef and ground pork, while occurring regularly in processed meat products such as cold cuts. Listeriosis can cause high fever, severe headache, neck stiffness, and nausea. Infections during pregnancy can lead to premature delivery, infection of the newborn, or even stillbirth.

Antibiotics

Another health problem associated with meat consumption stems from the intensive use of antibiotics in raising livestock. More than half of all antibiotics used in North America are administered to livestock, and in most cases antibiotics are used to accelerate growth, not treat infections. The inappropriate use of antibiotics in livestock is contributing to the growth of multidrug-resistant strains of bacteria, including *E. coli* O157:H7, *Salmonella,* and *Campylobacter,* and the spread of antibiotic-resistant organisms through the food supply. The U.S. Food and Drug Administration recently concluded that each year the use of fluoroquinolones in chickens compromises the treatment of almost ten thousand people who suffer from *Campylobacter* infections. When these people are treated with the fluoroquinolones commonly prescribed for *Campylobacter,* the bacteria are found to be resistant. Antibiotic resistance leads to more deaths and long-term illness from untreatable disease, increases the risk of drug-resistant pathogens spreading globally, and raises health care costs.

The inappropriate use of antibiotics in livestock is contributing to the growth of multidrug-resistant strains of bacteria

Hormones

Three natural hormones and three synthetically produced hormones are commonly given to cattle in Canada, the U.S., and Australia to make them gain weight faster. Scientists are concerned that these added hormones could affect the growth and development of children and may increase the risk of breast cancer. Another hormone called BGH (bovine growth hormone) is given to some dairy cows in the U.S., but is not allowed in Canada or Australia. BGH boosts milk production but causes inflammation and infection in cows, leading to treatment with antibiotics that could potentially end up in your milk.

Arsenic

Most of the billions of chickens and pigs raised in the U.S. and Canada are given feed that contains a form of arsenic to promote faster growth and kill parasites. While the form of arsenic fed to livestock is not hazardous, once ingested it is converted into highly toxic forms of arsenic.

A FOOD SAFETY PRIMER <<

Experts urge people to follow a handful of basic precautions to prevent exposure to foodborne pathogens:

> Keep clean. Always wash your hands thoroughly before preparing food and after going to the bathroom. Wash both hands for at least thirty seconds, front and back. Regularly wash all surfaces and equipment used in food preparation.

> Do not cross-contaminate. Separate raw meat, poultry, and seafood from other foods. Use separate knives and cutting boards for these products.

> Cook all foods thoroughly and at sufficiently high temperatures This applies especially to meat, poultry, seafood, and eggs.

> Keep food at safe temperatures. Do not keep cooked or perishable food at room temperature for more than two hours. Refrigerate or freeze cooked and perishable food. Do not thaw frozen food at room temperature.

> Eat safe foods. Do not consume food that has passed its expiry date.

Arsenic is a potent carcinogen. Chronic exposure can result in cancer of the skin, lung, bladder, and prostate. As well as finding its way into chicken meat, arsenic ends up in animal manure that is spread on farmland and absorbed by crops. Eventually some of this toxic substance leaches into groundwater.

WHAT YOU CAN DO

> Cut back on your consumption of meat, eggs, and dairy products. Choose leaner cuts and smaller portions, trim the fat, and limit meat to fewer weekly meals. Extensive evidence indicates that a diet with lower meat consumption will reduce your risk of various chronic diseases and lengthen life expectancy.

> Eat organic, grass-fed, and free-range meat, eggs, milk, and dairy products.

> Choose low-fat dairy products.

> Avoid hot dogs, bacon, cold cuts, and other processed meats. These meats are made with nitrates, which cooking can transform into nitrites and nitrosamines, both of which cause cancer. Charring meat increases the risk.

> Urge your government to catch up to world-leading practices in Europe. The use of antibiotics, growth hormones, and arsenic to accelerate the growth of livestock is prohibited in Europe because of concerns about harm to human health.

The Fish Counter

Fish is a healthy, highly nutritious food that provides protein and is low in saturated fat. Some species of fish contain high levels of omega-3 fatty acids, which are vital for pregnant women and young children because of their role in early brain development. However, the health benefits of eating fish must be weighed against serious concerns about toxic contaminants. Governments have issued fish consumption advisories warning individuals—especially pregnant or nursing women—to limit their intake of particular species of fish. The main concern is mercury, a potent neurotoxin that can harm the development of the fetus. Other contaminants of concern include dioxins and PCBs.

Contaminants

Mercury from human activities such as burning coal, garbage, and medical waste enters the atmosphere and eventually falls into water bodies where it is transformed into methyl mercury, a compound that accumulates in the food chain. This accumulation process means that a fish can have mercury levels thousands of times higher than the water it lives in. Usually, the larger and older the fish, the higher the mercury level. Both fresh water and marine fish are vulnerable to mercury contamination.

Both fresh water and marine fish are vulnerable to mercury contamination

Exposure of fetuses, infants, and young children to mercury, even at low levels, can cause a decrease in IQ, delays in walking and talking, lack of coordination, blindness, and seizures. Children whose mothers are exposed to elevated levels of mercury during pregnancy perform below average on neurological tests and lag behind in school. Hundreds of thousands of women of child-bearing age in the U.S., Canada, and Australia have mercury levels that pose a risk to their children. Mercury can also harm adults, causing reduced mental functioning and memory loss, infertility, tremors, changes in vision, deafness, loss of muscle coordination and sensation, and possibly diseases of the immune and cardiovascular systems. Eating fish, particularly large predatory species such as shark, swordfish, marlin, and some kinds of tuna, is the way most people are exposed to mercury.

PCBS were used in electric transformers for about fifty years until banned in the 1970s. Unfortunately, their toxic legacy continues because PCBS were carelessly dumped into the environment, contaminating rivers, lakes, and oceans. Like mercury, PCBs can interfere with brain development. Other adverse health effects include cancer and weakening of the immune system. Fish are the major dietary source of PCBs, but levels vary from species to species and from waterway to waterway. Research indicates that high levels of PCB contamination are found in farmed salmon, striped bass, and bluefish.

Shellfish are subject to contamination by both human activities and naturally occurring toxins such as paralytic shellfish poison. Along the coasts of Canada, the U.S., and Australia, thousands of square kilometers are subject to ongoing shellfish closures due to bacterial contamination from municipal waste water and other sources of pollution.

WHAT YOU CAN DO

> Unfortunately, the advice provided by governments is inconsistent. Although all governments agree that fish low in mercury can contribute to a healthy diet, they agree on little else. U.S. recommendations offer more protection to the most vulnerable people (women of childbearing age, pregnant women, nursing mothers, and young children), while Canada's recommendations offer more protection to the general public. Australia's fish consumption advice is weaker than the guidance provided in the U.S. and Canada. Consider this synthesis of the more health-protective elements of the Canadian and American warnings:

> Women who might become pregnant, women who are pregnant, nursing mothers, and young children should avoid eating fresh or frozen tuna, shark, swordfish, escolar, marlin, king mackerel, tilefish, and orange roughy.

> Everyone else should limit consumption of these fish (all species combined) to a maximum of 150 grams (5 ounces) per week.

> Canned albacore or white tuna has more mercury than canned light tuna. Women who might become pregnant, women who are pregnant, and nursing mothers should limit themselves to one average meal of albacore tuna—170 grams (6 ounces)—per week.

> Parents should follow these recommendations when feeding fish and shellfish to young children, but serve smaller portions.

> Be cautious about eating fish that you catch in local waters. First, check with local, provincial, or state environmental health agencies to learn if there are fish consumption advisories in your area. Second, choose species and sizes of fish that are less likely to be contaminated (avoid large, older fish and bottom feeders). Third, carefully clean and cook your fish, discarding fatty parts. Fourth, if no advice about fish safety is available, limit yourself to one average meal of fish from local waters—170 grams (6 ounces)—per week, and do not consume any other fish during that week.

> Choose fish with high levels of omega-3 fatty acids and low levels of mercury, such as anchovy, capelin, char, herring, Atlantic mackerel, mullet, wild salmon (not farmed salmon), smelt, rainbow trout, lake whitefish, blue crab, shrimp, clam, mussel, and oyster.

> Trim fatty portions of fish to reduce exposure to dioxins and PCBs (fat is where these substances are stored). Mercury is stored in muscle tissue and thus can't be removed by trimming.

> Choose fish that has been caught or raised sustainably. In the U.S., see www.seafoodwatch.org and www.ewg.org for up-to-date advice. In Canada, see www.seachoice.org. In Australia, see www.amcs.org.au.

> Consider adding plant-based sources of omega-3 fatty acids to your diet, such as flaxseed oil, canola oil, soybeans, soybean oil, pumpkin seeds, pumpkin seed oil, purslane, perilla seed oil, walnuts, and walnut oil. Although not a perfect substitute, plant-based omega-3 fatty acids can be converted by most people's bodies into the coveted type present in seafood.

The Fresh Produce Section

Fruits and vegetables are a vital part of a healthy diet, and most people need to eat more of them in order to meet nutritional guidelines. Diets rich in fresh fruits and vegetables reduce the risk of cancers and are linked to longer life expectancy. However, there are two types of environmental hazards associated with fresh produce: pesticide residues and pathogens. There is also an ongoing controversy about genetically modified foods, which are not identified or labeled as such and are thus indistinguishable from their conventional counterparts.

Pesticides

Today's agricultural pesticides are less of a danger to human health than pesticides used in the past because they are generally less toxic, less persistent, and less likely to keep on accumulating in living organisms and the environment. However, "less dangerous" is not the same as "safe." Light cigarettes are less dangerous than regular cigarettes but still cause cancer. Hundreds of commercial pesticides formerly manufactured and promoted by industry and deemed safe by governments have been banned because of evidence that they caused health and environmental damage. It is almost certain that we will continue to make disturbing discoveries about the adverse effects of today's pesticides.

> It is almost certain that we will continue to make disturbing discoveries about the adverse effects of today's pesticides

Pesticide exposures can produce two types of adverse health effects—acute, short-term effects and chronic, long-term effects. Acute pesticide poisoning can affect the eyes, skin, nervous system, respiratory system, cardiovascular system, and gastrointestinal tract. Back in 1985, an insecticide called aldicarb was improperly used on watermelons, causing more than a thousand people in the U.S. and Canada to become ill. Thankfully, episodes of acute pesticide poisoning caused by the consumption of fresh fruits and vegetables are rare today.

The chronic health effects of pesticide exposures can include increased risk of cancer (e.g., non-Hodgkin's lymphoma and childhood leukemia), neurological impairment (e.g., Parkinson's disease, Alzheimer's disease), developmental damage, reproductive problems, organ damage, and interference with the human hormone system. In 2006, a study published in the *Annals of Neurology* looked at the relationship between pesticide exposure and Parkinson's disease in over 140,000 people. Exposure to pesticides increased the likelihood that an individual would suffer from Parkinson's disease by 70%. Another recent study found that individuals exposed to substantial quantities of pesticides face triple the risk of non-Hodgkin's lymphoma that unexposed individuals face. There is still uncertainty about the long-term effects of exposure to low levels of multiple pesticides, and the combined effects of exposure to pesticides and other toxic substances. The most vulnerable people are farmers and agricultural workers.

Europe has banned many pesticides that are still used in North America and Australia

Government tests demonstrate that blueberries and celery may be contaminated with up to thirteen different pesticide residues. A single grapefruit, orange, or melon may have residues from up to six different pesticides, fresh peas and snow peas (from China) seven, and a sweet bell pepper (from Mexico) as many as nine. Pesticide residues detected on Mexican sweet bell peppers include endosulfan, metalaxyl, and permethrin—pesticides banned by the European Union because of their health and environmental effects. Overall, testing by the U.S. Department of Agriculture detected pesticide residues on 77% of fresh fruits and vegetables and 40% of processed fruits and vegetables, although less than 1% of these tests revealed residues above legal limits. In Canada, government testing found pesticide residues on only 10% of produce tested. However, it would be misleading to think that Canadian produce is safer, since Canada employs a less rigorous approach to testing for pesticides.

Overall, governments in Canada, the U.S., and Australia do less to protect public health and the environment from the adverse effects of pesticides than their European counterparts. Based on health and environmental concerns, Europe has banned many pesticides that are still used in North America and Australia. An example is atrazine, a pesticide that contaminates groundwater and can impair the sexual development of frogs, turning them into hermaphrodites at concentrations similar to those found in some Canadian, American, and Australian drinking water. Europe banned all uses of atrazine in 2004. Canada also allows pesticide residues on some fruits and vegetables at levels that are up to fourteen hundred times higher than permissible in Europe.

Foodborne Pathogens
Fresh produce can also be a source of pathogens, including bacteria such as *Listeria monocytogenes, Salmonella, Shigella,* and *E. Coli* O157: H7, and viruses such as hepatitis A. Food contaminated by bacteria or viruses may not look or smell spoiled. The risk of bacterial contamination is greater in some produce and related products:

- Sprouts. These can be contaminated by *E. coli* bacteria that enter the sprout seed and multiply in the warm and humid sprouting conditions.

- Lettuce and fresh herbs. These difficult-to-wash plants are grown close to the ground where they can come in contact with pathogens.

- Fresh-cut vegetables. When the skin of fruits and vegetables is cut, bacteria can enter and contaminate the fresh-cut and packaged product.

- Tomatoes. These can be contaminated in fields or packing houses as a result of poor sanitary conditions.

- Melons. The skin of melons, particularly the grooved skin of cantaloupe, can harbor bacteria that contaminate the fruit when it is cut.

- Berries. With their soft skins and irregular surfaces, fresh berries are vulnerable to bacterial contamination. Raspberries are especially susceptible because of their covering of tiny hairs.

- Unpasteurized juices and prepared salads (coleslaw, potato salad, pasta salad, and fruit salad). These products should be handled with care.

While most cases of foodborne illness involve products of animal origin, fruits and vegetables do present some risk. As well as the concerns already described, two others are worth mentioning: the viruses that can contaminate food touched by infected food handlers, and the toxins produced by many species of mushrooms. Depending on the type and quantity ingested, mushrooms can have severe effects. Victims of mushroom poisoning usually mistake a toxic variety for a safe variety.

Genetically Modified Foods

Humans have been altering plants and animals to produce food for thousands of years. The sheep raised today for fleece and meat are descended from animals first domesticated in ancient Mesopotamia. Broccoli, brussels sprouts, and cabbage all trace their origins to a single species of mustard. Genetically modified (GM) foods, however, are distinct in two key ways: GM organisms do not result from generations of breeding but from inserting genes directly into an existing organism to create an immediate change; and the new genes inserted in a GM organism can come from any plant, animal, or microbe. For example, a fish gene can be inserted into a tomato plant to improve cold weather tolerance.

GM foods have several potential benefits. They could result in higher crop yields, enabling us to feed more people. They might also require less use of pesticides and other toxic substances, and might permit the addition of essential nutrients to crops. For example, efforts are now underway to genetically modify rice so that it contains vitamin A, which could help remedy a chronic deficiency affecting 400 million people worldwide. Whether these anticipated benefits will actually be realized remains unclear, as studies have produced conflicting results about GM crops, yields, and pesticide use.

GM foods also present potential risks to human health. Some research suggests that GM foods may cause allergic reactions, contribute to nutritional deficiencies, or inflict damage on organs and the immune system. Crops used to produce drugs could inadvertently contaminate regular crops with these pharmaceutical products. Human error and unpredictable natural conditions make this kind of contamination likely. The use of antibiotic-resistant genes in GM crops could exacerbate problems with antibiotic resistance. Another worry is that toxic substances or allergens could be produced through the genetic modification process. A chemical that is widely used in treating GM crops, glyphosate (used in the commercial product Roundup) may be an endocrine disruptor, causing problems in human reproduction. Food safety and food security could also be affected by outcrossing—the movement of genes from GM plants into conventional crops or related species in the wild—as well as the mixing of crops derived from conventional seeds with those grown using GM crops. Traces of a corn type only approved for feed use have already appeared in corn products destined for human consumption in the U.S. The bottom line is that we do not know about the long-term health effects of producing and eating genetically modified foods.

WHAT YOU CAN DO

> Buy organic food, especially if you have children (see page 91). If you can't afford to go completely organic, focus your efforts on baby food, meat, dairy products, peaches, apples, sweet bell peppers, celery, nectarines, strawberries, cherries, lettuce, grapes, pears, spinach, and potatoes. These products are more likely to be contaminated with pesticides and other harmful substances if they are not produced organically. However, because fresh fruits and vegetables play such a vital role in promoting and protecting our health, you should not cut back on the amount you consume in order to eat organic produce.

> Buy local produce. Tests indicate that imported produce is twice as likely to violate rules governing maximum pesticide residue levels. Local produce is also likely to be fresher.

> Thoroughly rinse produce with tap water and ignore attempts to sell you special cleaning solutions. They are a waste of money.

> Grow your own food, either in your own yard, on your balcony, or in a community garden. The rewards for getting your hands dirty will include delicious vegetables, fruits, and fresh herbs as well as heightened appreciation for farmers and a closer connection to your local environment.

> Urge your government to require labeling of genetically modified foods. Labeling is not required in Canada, the U.S., or Australia despite overwhelming public support for this.

The Processed Food Aisles

The inner aisles of grocery stores are packed with a dazzling array of processed foods—candy, salty snacks, sugary drinks, breakfast cereals, meal replacement bars, and countless other packaged foods. Most processed foods depend on a range of food additives and artificial colors.

Additives

Food additives include preservatives, artificial flavors, emulsifiers, thickeners, stabilizers, anti-caking agents, and sweeteners. Health concerns related to food additives include allergies, cancer, and adverse effects on the behavior of children. For example, monosodium glutamate (MSG) is added to food to enhance natural flavors, but some individuals who are sensitive to MSG may experience a burning sensation in the chest, neck, abdomen, or extremities, facial pressure, headache, nausea, and chest pains. Aspartame (Nutrasweet), Acesulfame-K (Ace-K), and saccharin are artificial sweeteners used in many diet foods, including desserts, drinks, chewing gum, and baked goods. There is conflicting evidence regarding their safety for human consumption. Olestra is a fat substitute with no calories that is used in some chips and crackers. It passes through the digestive system intact (explaining why it has no calories) but causes gastrointestinal problems, including cramps, bloating, flatulence, and diarrhea.

ORGANIC FOOD OFFERS health and environmental benefits, including lower risks associated with pesticide exposure for both farmers and consumers. When people switch their diets from food grown with pesticides to organic food, pesticide residues in their urine quickly drop to undetectable levels. Evidence suggests that organic food is more nutritious than conventional food, offering higher levels of vitamins and minerals (calcium, iron, magnesium). Some organic crops contain higher levels of antioxidants and polyphenols that may help prevent cardiovascular disease and cancer. A recent review of nearly a hundred studies concluded that the nutritional premium of organic food averaged 25%.

As well as being better for our health, organic agriculture is much better for the environment. The methods used by organic farmers require fewer nonrenewable resources, have less impact on wildlife, prevent water contamination, and avoid soil degradation.

Diacetyl is a chemical used to enhance the flavor of microwave popcorn. It's responsible for a devastating lung disease that primarily affects workers in facilities that produce microwave popcorn. Sodium nitrate and nitrite are added to meats to give them their red color and provide smoked flavor. These additives mix with stomach acid to form nitrosamines, which can cause cancer. BHA (butylated hydroxyanisole) and BHT (butylated hydroxytoluene) are preservatives that prevent rancidity in oils and foods containing oils. The U.S. Department of Health and Human Services describes BHA as "reasonably anticipated to be a human carcinogen based on sufficient evidence of carcinogenicity in experimental animals."

> Three out of four people consume levels of salt—mostly from processed foods—far in excess of what doctors recommend

Despite the disturbing adverse health effects associated with food additives, it is worth remembering that a far larger number of people are harmed by two familiar substances routinely added to food: salt and sugar. Three out of four people consume levels of salt—mostly from processed foods—far in excess of what doctors recommend. Reducing salt intake can lower blood pressure and reduce the risk of cardiovascular disease by 25%. The average American consumes more than 60 kilograms (132 pounds) of sugar and related sweeteners annually, contributing significantly to the obesity epidemic. Even seemingly healthy foods are implicated. For example, yogurt and breakfast cereals are often more like desserts because they contain so much added sugar.

Artificial Colors

Artificial colors, often made from coal tar or petroleum, are in a wide range of processed foods, including candy, cold cuts, hot dogs, sausages, soft drinks, sports drinks, fruit juices, breakfast cereals, children's snacks, and baked goods. Nine food dyes are approved for use in the U.S.: Brilliant Blue FCF (Blue 1), Citrus Red No. 2, Indigotine (Blue 2), Fast Green FCF (Green 3), Orange B, Erythrosine (Red 3), Allura Red (Red 40),

Tartrazine (Yellow 5), and Sunset Yellow FCF (Yellow 6). Orange B, used in the U.S. only for hot dog and sausage casings, is not allowed in Canada. Canada allows the use of two additional artificial colors, Amaranth (Red 2) and Ponseau SX. Australia allows the use of fourteen artificial colors, including five not used in the U.S. or Canada. Amaranth (Red 2) is a suspected carcinogen and has been banned in the U.S. since 1976. In both Canada and the U.S., Citrus Red No. 2 is limited to use on the peel of oranges because it is a possible human carcinogen. Fast Green FCF (Green 3) is already banned in Europe because of links to bladder cancer. Hundreds of thousands of people have allergic reactions to Tartrazine (Yellow 5).

There is a growing body of research linking the consumption of food dyes to attention deficit hyperactivity disorder in children. The British Food Standards Agency advises parents that children exhibiting these behavioral problems should avoid foods containing artificial colors. Based on recent scientific research, the European Union is in the process of banning artificial colors in food. However, governments in the U.S., Canada, and Australia continue to deny that there is a problem.

WHAT YOU CAN DO

> Eat whole foods—fruits, vegetables, grains, nuts, seeds, beans, and legumes that have not been extensively refined or processed. Whole foods offer higher nutritional value and protection from health problems like obesity, diabetes, cancer, and cardiovascular disease. Nutritionists remind us to consider a simple rule—the more processed a food, the lower its nutritional value is likely to be.

> Read food labels, and avoid products containing artificial colors, artificial sweeteners, fat substitutes, MSG, diacetyl, BHA, BHT, sodium nitrate, aluminum, and nitrite. The Center for Science in the Public Interest offers information on food additives at www.cspinet.org/reports/chemcuisine. htm.

> Reduce consumption of processed foods containing added salt and other types of sodium. Also reduce consumption of foods containing added sugar and other types of sweeteners, including high fructose corn syrup, glucose, and dextrose.

> Avoid products with long lists of ingredients you don't recognize and can't pronounce. If you need a degree in biochemistry to decipher the ingredients, odds are the food product is bad for you and the environment.

Advice for Parents

A healthy diet gives your children the opportunity to fulfill their potential and live a long, active life. Protect your children's health by taking these steps:

> Follow the longstanding advice of nutrition experts and feed your children a diverse diet of fresh, wholesome foods, plenty of fruits and vegetables, a variety of different protein sources, and the occasional treat.

> Make sure your children get plenty of fresh air and exercise, to prevent them from becoming overweight or obese.

> Feed your children organic food whenever possible. See the priority foods identified in the earlier section on organics, and avoid nonorganic fruit leather and fruit bars—a Canadian government study found pesticide residues on a majority of these products. The pesticides detected included thiabendazole (banned in Denmark and Slovenia), carbaryl (banned in Austria, Germany, and Sweden), and diphenylamine.

> Avoid foods containing artificial colors—especially if your children suffer from attention deficit hyperactivity disorder.

> Pregnant women should take additional precautions by avoiding high-risk foods:

> · Non-dried deli meats, including cold cuts, hot dogs, and smoked salmon.

- Undercooked meat, poultry, and seafood.
- Raw milk and dairy products, including soft and semi-soft cheeses such as Brie or Camembert.
- Raw sprouts, especially alfalfa sprouts.
- Fish containing high levels of mercury.
- Raw fish, especially shellfish such as oysters and clams.
- Foods made with raw or lightly cooked eggs, such as home-made Caesar salad dressing.
- Unpasteurized juices and apple cider.

Wrap-up

Today's diets are an unmitigated disaster from both health and environmental perspectives. Yet eating a diet that's good for both people and the planet is pretty simple. The succinct advice at the beginning of this chapter from author Michael Pollan says it all: "Eat food, not too much, mostly plants." By "food" Pollan means whole foods, not processed food, fast food, or junk food. His phrase "not too much" underscores the importance of reducing our caloric intake to prevent obesity. Eating fewer calories will also reduce our exposure to all of the environmental hazards encountered in the food system. And when he says "mostly plants," he reminds us to consume less meat. Eating less and eating lower on the food chain means that we will save money and can afford to boost the quality of the food we eat. While many people concerned about environmental hazards in the food supply tend to focus on pesticides, experts believe that persistent organic pollutants, heavy metals, and foodborne pathogens pose more significant health risks. Therefore it makes sense to focus your efforts on avoiding these contaminants.

Eating less and eating lower on the food chain means that we will save money and can afford to boost the quality of the food we eat

A healthy diet for humans is also healthy for the planet. The livestock industry produces more climate-changing greenhouse gas emissions than the global transportation system. Organic agriculture produces comparable volumes of healthier food on a given area of land but with a much smaller environmental footprint. Wholesome, local foods require less packaging, processing, and shipping, saving energy and reducing greenhouse gas emissions, chemical use, and waste. Plus local foods taste better. Reducing your intake of junk food, fast food, and other highly processed foods will reduce your ecological footprint and improve your health.

Eat Healthy Food

> If you are overweight or obese, make a concerted effort to eat fewer calories.

> Wash your hands frequently and keep food preparation areas clean.

> Cut back on your consumption of meat, eggs, and dairy products, and choose low-fat, organic options when you do eat these foods.

> Select fish that is high in omega-3 fatty acids and low in contaminants.

> Eat lots of local, organic fruits and vegetables.

> Focus on whole foods and avoid potentially harmful additives.

5 THE WATER WE DRINK

I never drink water because of the disgusting things that fish do in it.
W.C. Fields

TWO HYDROGEN ATOMS and one oxygen atom gives us H_2O. Just as we depend on air and food, we depend on water for a wide range of physiological functions and processes. Over the course of a month, healthy people will replace every molecule of water in their bodies with fresh water molecules. Our kidneys filter approximately 175 liters (46 gallons) of blood daily, sending out waste and contaminants in urine and feces. If we are deprived of water for a few days, dehydration from urinating, sweating, breathing, and defecating will gradually reduce the volume of our blood and trigger a series of responses culminating in unconsciousness and, eventually, death.

Life on Earth began in water, more than 4 billion years ago, and to this day every known form of life is dependent upon water. This explains why some scientists are so excited about finding water on Mars. Water covers about 70% of the Earth's surface and makes up roughly the same proportion of our bodies. While your bones may consist of only 33% water, your brain may consist of 85% water. As Dr. David Suzuki wrote in *The Sacred Balance,* "Basically, each of us is a blob of water with enough macro-molecular thickening to give us some stiffness and keep us from dribbling away." By comparison, a jellyfish is approximately 95% water.

Incredibly, we can access only 0.01% of the world's water supply for human use, with the rest located in salty oceans, polar ice and glaciers, or caverns deep underground. Despite its extraordinary value, we treat water in much the same way we treat the atmosphere—as a place where society can dump unwanted refuse, including industrial chemicals, pharmaceuticals such as antibiotics, mood stabilizers, and sex hormones, and untreated or inadequately treated sewage. Hundreds of millions of kilograms of industrial pollutants and pesticides, billions of kilograms of manure and fertilizers, contamination from millions of boats, and immense volumes of urban runoff find their way into our water bodies. In Canada and the U.S., industries dump over 800,000 kilograms (more than 1.5 million pounds) of known or suspected carcinogens—including lead, chloroform, and carbon tetrachloride—into rivers, lakes, and other water bodies every year. In addition, more than 16 million kilograms (35 million pounds) of known or suspected carcinogens are injected underground where they may contaminate water supplies. We need to recognize that the pollutants dumped into water bodies or buried in soil and rock are likely to end up in our bodies. This insight should lead to greater respect for water.

> We treat water in much the same way we treat the atmosphere—as a place where society can dump unwanted refuse

In today's world, water in rivers, lakes, and streams is never "pure." Seemingly pristine water bodies—such as lakes high in the Rocky Mountains—can still be contaminated with everything from prohibited pesticides carried north on air currents to parasites such as *Giardia* transmitted by wildlife. Regardless of where it comes from, surface water should always be disinfected before drinking.

More and more people who are concerned about the health effects, taste, odor, or color of their drinking water are taking action. One in two Canadian households and two in five American households report using a home filtration system of some kind. A growing number of people have turned to bottled water. In Canada, a country internationally renowned for its abundant fresh water, almost three in ten families depend primarily on bottled water. One in five Americans drinks only bottled water. These people are paying up to a thousand times the cost of municipal tap water for a product that may offer them zero health benefits. Equally absurd is the fact that Canada and the U.S. import bottled water from far-flung locales such as Fiji, Europe, and even Ethiopia.

Health Hazards in Drinking Water

The provision of safe drinking water to the majority of the world's population is one of the great public health achievements of recent centuries. However, it would be a mistake to take drinking water for granted, even in wealthy nations, despite a plethora of laws, policies, programs, and public infrastructure investments. In Canada, the U.S., and Australia, a number of high-profile water contamination events have occurred in recent years. In 2000, seven people died, sixty-five were hospitalized, and thousands more became ill when the water supply of Walkerton, Ontario, was contaminated with *E. coli* O157:H7. The Canadian government estimates that contaminated drinking water causes an estimated ninety deaths and ninety thousand cases of illness annually, although it acknowledges major data gaps and widespread under-reporting of waterborne disease. In the U.S., the worst waterborne disease outbreak in recent history occurred in Milwaukee, Wisconsin, in 1993. Caused by the protozoa *Cryptosporidium,* this public health crisis resulted in more than 50 deaths, 4,400 hospitalizations, and more than 400,000 cases of illness. Clusters of childhood cancer cases in Woburn, Massachusetts, and Dover Township, New Jersey, are blamed on contaminated drinking water consumed by pregnant women from the 1960s to the 1990s. In both communities, the water contained high levels of trichloroethylene and other solvents. Experts estimate that contaminated drinking water in the U.S. may cause up to 1,200 deaths, 4.2 million to 32.8 million cases of acute gastrointestinal illness (the wide range indicates the level of uncertainty), and an unknown number of cases of other diseases annually. The most widely publicized incident of drinking water contamination in Australia occurred in 1998 in Sydney. High numbers of *Cryptosporidium* and *Giardia* organisms were discovered in municipally treated water, and boil water advisories were issued for 3 million residents.

Consumption of drinking water that contains pathogens (disease-causing microorganisms) or contaminants (chemical, physical, and radiological) results in a wide range of negative effects on human health. Waterborne pathogens such as bacteria, viruses, and protozoa can cause disease outbreaks that result in acute health problems for large numbers of people. Diarrhea, abdominal cramps, vomiting, headaches, and fever can occur within hours or days of consuming contaminated water. Most people can fight off the infections that cause these symptoms and experience no permanent ill effects. However, waterborne pathogens can be dangerous or even deadly for a person whose immune system is already weak because of chemotherapy, steroid use, an organ transplant, or HIV/AIDS.

In contrast, chemical and radiological contaminants cause chronic health problems that generally arise after prolonged periods of exposure. Examples of these chronic effects include cancer, liver or kidney problems, and reproductive difficulties. While food and air are more likely sources of exposure to chemical contaminants than drinking water, lead, nitrates, arsenic, and disinfection by-products in water pose a substantial health risk.

Microbiological Contaminants

Experts agree that the greatest risks from consuming drinking water in industrialized nations are posed by microbiological contaminants. The three main categories of these waterborne pathogens are bacteria (e.g., *E. coli* O157:H7, *Salmonella*, *Shigella*, and *Campylobacter*), viruses (e.g., hepatitis A), and protozoa (e.g., *Giardia*, *Cryptosporidium*, and *Toxoplasma*). Surface water is most at risk of microbiological contamination by wildlife and human activities. However, groundwater (from wells) is at more risk than previously thought, due to secondary contamination from polluted surface waters. The adverse effects caused by waterborne pathogens range from mild gastroenteritis (upset stomach) to severe diarrhea and death. Those most likely to be infected and suffer serious adverse health effects are infants, young children, people with compromised immune systems, and the elderly.

Chemical Contaminants

Potential health effects associated with exposure to chemicals in drinking water include cancer, neurological disorders, gastrointestinal illness, reproductive problems, and disruption of the hormone system. The majority of harmful chemicals found in water are caused by human activities. Pesticides, fertilizers, hydrocarbons, and solvents are major concerns. As well, toxic metals can leach into water supplies from sources ranging from mines to plumbing. Some harmful substances, such as arsenic, can occur naturally in drinking water supplies.

A significant health concern related to public drinking water involves disinfection by-products such as trihalomethanes and haloacetic acids. These are created when a substance used for disinfecting drinking water (typically chlorine) interacts with substances that occur naturally in the water supply. Disinfection by-products are linked to bladder, colon, and other cancers, as well as increased rates of miscarriage. Most experts believe that these cancer risks are smaller than the health risks posed by pathogens in water that is not disinfected. In other words, despite the dangers posed by disinfection, the benefits outweigh the risks. Fortunately, you can protect your health from disinfection by-products and reduce your risk of cancer by using an activated carbon filter (see "Filtration," page 107). As well, there are actions that water suppliers can take

Disinfection by-products are linked to bladder, colon, and other cancers, as well as increased rates of miscarriage

to reduce or eliminate the risk posed by disinfection by-products. These include limiting organic materials in the source water and disinfecting water with ultraviolet radiation.

Radiological Contaminants

Radiological contaminants in drinking water include naturally occurring substances such as uranium and radon, as well as a wide range of radionuclides resulting from human activities, including mining, the operation of nuclear reactors, and the disposal of nuclear waste. The acute health effects of radiation—burns, vomiting, reduced white blood cell counts—occur at high exposures and are not caused by drinking water. Exposure to radiation at low doses over a long time, however, is linked to increased risks of cancer and genetic disorders. Drinking water contaminated with radionuclides causes internal exposure to radiation that can last for months or even years. The radiation dose resulting from ingestion depends on a number of biological and chemical factors. Health effects depend on the type of radiation and the tissues or organs that are exposed. The good news is that generally less than 10% of human exposure to radiation comes from drinking water. However, if your indoor air contains high levels of radon and you rely on well water, you should have your water tested for radon and install a treatment system if levels are high.

The good news is that generally less than 10% of human exposure to radiation comes from drinking water

How to Minimize Your Risk

You can take two steps to address concerns about environmental hazards in your drinking water. Whether your water comes from a public system or a private source, the steps are the same:

> Find out what is in your water.

> Take remedial action if necessary.

In addition, you can take the very important step of acting to protect water bodies from pollution.

Find Out What Is in Your Water

It is essential to learn where your water comes from, what kind of treatment (if any) it receives, and what contaminants may be in the water flowing from your tap. You face different kinds of risks depending on whether your water comes from a large public system, a small public system (serving up to a few thousand people), or a private source such as a well (see page 105). There are two main differences between publicly supplied water and privately supplied water. First, public water supplies, are almost always treated prior to distribution and consumption. Second, public water supplies are regularly monitored for water quality. In contrast, few regulations govern the quality of private water supplies, and testing is up to the owner. Small public systems face higher risks than large public systems because they operate with fewer resources, less monitoring, and weaker regulations. If you rely on a small public system, you may wish to follow the testing advice for private water supplies.

If you are served by a public utility, find out about the contaminants that may be in your water supply. Throughout the U.S. and in an increasing number of Canadian provinces, regulations require public water suppliers to send all customers an annual water quality report (often called a Consumer Confidence Report). These reports offer useful information about the source of your water, levels of contaminants, levels at which these contaminants are a health concern, and violations of any rules related to drinking water quality. If you are not receiving these reports, call the water supplier named on your utility bill. Most communities also publish their drinking water quality reports on the Internet. A comprehensive listing for American communities is available at www.epa.gov/safewater/dwinfo/index.html.

Water quality reports do not provide the complete picture, however, because they describe the water being pumped into the distribution system, not the water emerging from your tap. Drinking water can pick up contaminants—most importantly lead—in the distribution system or in your plumbing. Therefore, testing for lead may be a good idea (see "Lead," page 113).

If you rely on a private source, such as a well, river, or lake, have your water tested annually for total coliform bacteria, nitrates, total dissolved solids, and pH levels. If you have reason to suspect other contaminants (e.g., pesticides from a nearby farm or contaminants from a nearby gas station), you can also test for these. Many serious problems—bacteria, heavy metals, and nitrates—can only be found by laboratory testing of water. Always use a certified laboratory, which you can find in the Yellow Pages or on the Internet. In the U.S., call the Safe Drinking Water hotline 1-800-426-4791 or visit www.epa.gov/safewater/labs/index.html. Depending on how many contaminants you test for, a water quality test can cost twenty dollars or hundreds of dollars. It's a good investment in your health.

Testing more than once a year may be warranted in the following circumstances:

- Someone in your household is pregnant or nursing.
- Household members are experiencing unexplained illnesses.
- Your neighbors have found a dangerous contaminant in their water.
- You have noted a change in water taste, odor, color, or clarity.
- A spill of chemicals or fuels has occurred into or near your well.
- You have replaced or repaired a part of your well system.

The best time to sample water from a well, river, or lake is when the probability of contamination is highest. This is likely to be after the ground thaws in early spring, after an extended dry spell, after heavy rains, or after the source has not been used for lengthy periods. You should continue to monitor the quality of your water at least annually, whether or not you choose to use a home water treatment system.

THE RISK OF having problems depends on where your well is located and how it is built and maintained. It also depends on your local environment—the quality of the source from which you draw your water and the local activities that could contaminate it. The following steps will help you maintain the safety of your well water:

> Hire a certified well driller for any new well construction or modification.

> Install a locking well cap or sanitary seal to prevent unauthorized use of, or entry into, the well.

> Keep potential sources of contamination (pesticides, fertilizers, used oil, fuels) away from the area. Don't put anything on the ground that you don't want to drink.

> Maintain your septic system properly—pump out the tank regularly and prevent trees from growing on top of the septic field.

> Have your water tested annually for coliform bacteria, nitrates, and other contaminants.

> Perform maintenance on your well regularly. This may include testing the flow rate, checking the water level, and inspecting the pump motor.

> Keep accurate, up-to-date records (construction contract or report, maintenance, disinfection, water testing results).

> Take immediate action to remedy any problems that arise.

> For further information, check the U.S. Environmental Protection Agency's excellent website on private wells at www.epa.gov/safewater/privatewells/index2.html.

Take Remedial Action If Necessary

After your drinking water has been analyzed, compare the levels of contaminants found with those listed in government regulations. The presence of contaminants in drinking water is generally not cause for alarm. What matters is the level or concentration of a particular contaminant relative to established standards.

If any contaminants in your water exceed recommended levels, immediate action is required. Even if contaminants exceed half of the standard, you may wish to take preventive or precautionary action because some drinking water rules are based not only on health considerations but also on the cost of treatment. For example, current standards for arsenic and disinfection by-products expose individuals to a higher risk of cancer than governments usually deem acceptable because the cost of dealing with these substances is perceived to be too expensive.

While the primary reason for taking remedial action is to remove specific contaminants revealed by testing, you may also take action to:

> Protect a member of your household who has a compromised immune system because of age, illness, or a specific health condition.

> Improve the taste or odor of your water.

> Address staining problems.

Once you've decided that action is required to improve or safeguard your water quality, you'll need to choose between various home water treatment systems and bottled water. If your only concern is to improve the taste or odor of your drinking water, a simple activated carbon filter may be all that you need (see "Filtration," page 107). If your goal is to address health concerns, a little more research into the two main options—treatment devices and bottled water—will be required to identify the right approach.

Water Treatment Devices

The choice of a home water treatment system will depend on the particular contaminants found in your water supply and the type of home you live in (detached house versus condominium or apartment). No single technology is currently capable of addressing all potential drinking water problems. One basic distinction is between point-of-use (pitcher or kitchen tap) devices and point-of-entry (whole house) devices. Point-of-use devices are portable, plumbed-in, or mounted on a faucet, and are used to treat water for drinking and cooking. Point-of-entry devices are installed on the main water supply line and treat all the water entering the building. Two point-of-entry water treatment devices widely used in rural areas are water softeners and greensand filters. These devices cannot provide adequate protection from pathogens or chemicals, although they may be useful in conjunction with other water treatment devices.

> No single technology is currently capable of addressing all potential drinking water problems

If you decide to use a home water treatment device, it is important to install, operate, and maintain it according to the manufacturer's instructions. In addition, it's a good idea to test the treated water several times throughout the first year of operation to ensure the system is working properly.

Filtration

All filtration systems filter water through screens with microscopic holes, measured in microns. When comparing filters, look for an absolute rating (the largest hole) not a nominal rating (the average hole). In general, protozoa are removed by filters with an absolute rating of 1.0 micron, bacteria by 0.1 micron, and viruses by 0.01 micron. The smaller the hole size, the cleaner the water will be. Filters, depending on their type, can remove a range of chemicals, including pesticides, industrial solvents, PCBs, and polycyclic aromatic hydrocarbons. An activated carbon filter will remove disinfection by-products linked to cancer and reproductive problems. Filtration generally does not remove calcium and magnesium—the minerals that make water "hard"—or sodium, nitrates, and fluoride. Specific types of filters are needed to remove bacteria, viruses, lead, and other heavy metals.

Various options are available for point-of-use filtration, including pitchers, faucet units, countertop units, and under-sink units. Because models of these and point-of-entry systems change so often, it is best to consult the NSF (National Sanitation Foundation) at www.nsf.org or Consumer Reports at www.ConsumerReports.org.

An activated carbon filter will remove disinfection by-products linked to cancer and reproductive problems

Note that chemicals such as bisphenol A may leach into stored water from the plastic used in some pitcher-style systems, and that the activated carbon filters used in many water treatment devices are a potential source of contamination. Over time, filters can become saturated with chemical contaminants and release these substances into the treated water. As well, the buildup of organic matter on a filter can lead to bacterial growth. For these reasons, filter cartridges should be changed on a regular basis as recommended by the manufacturer (usually after a specified number of months or volume of water treated). Be sure to choose a certified replacement cartridge. Water not consumed immediately after treatment should always be stored in the refrigerator to avoid microbial contamination.

Other Options

In a reverse osmosis system, pressure forces water through a semi-permeable membrane that captures certain contaminants. Reverse osmosis is used to reduce high levels of nitrates, heavy metals, sulfate, sodium, and total dissolved solids. Some, but not all, reverse osmosis systems are effective in dealing with bacteria and disinfection by-products. Reverse osmosis uses a lot of water, with 75% to 90% of water that enters the system being discharged as wastewater. These systems require regular monitoring and maintenance.

In a distillation system, water is boiled and then the steam is condensed into purer water. Distillation is used to soften water and to remove nitrates, bacteria, sodium, dissolved solids, organic compounds, heavy metals, and radionuclides. Some distillers are not effective for volatile organic compounds (VOCs) and certain pesticides. Distillers are expensive to purchase and operate, and have limited capacity.

In an ultraviolet light system, UV radiation is used to kill microorganisms found in drinking water, including bacteria, viruses, and protozoa. UV treatment does not remove chlorine, VOCs, heavy metals, or other chemical contaminants and is only suitable when concerns are limited to microbiological contaminants.

Bottled Water

The alternative to a home water treatment system is bottled water. There is a raging debate about whether bottled water is better for your health than tap water. In many countries, different laws and regulations apply to drinking water than to bottled water. Experts suggest that the rules governing bottled water are weaker and point to the quality problems experienced by some bottled water suppliers. Bottled water generally comes from the same sources as tap water, but undergoes extra filtering or other treatment steps. In fact, a large proportion of bottled water is simply municipal tap water that has undergone additional treatment.

Does this additional treatment make bottled water safer? Not necessarily. A study published in the *Archives of Family Medicine* found that fifteen of fifty-seven bottled water samples bought in Cleveland, Ohio, had bacterial counts at least twice as high as Cleveland's tap water. The highest had more than a thousand times the amount of bacteria found in any of the tap water samples. A test of bottled water by the Environmental Working Group found levels of cancer-causing trihalomethanes exceeding legal limits in several samples as well as detectable levels of the pain-relieving medication acetaminophen, caffeine, arsenic, radioactive isotopes, nitrates, ammonia, degreasing agents, and solvents. Similarly, the Natural Resources Defense Council found contaminants in 20% of the bottled water they tested, including styrene, toluene, xylene, arsenic, and bacteria. A Canadian study found samples of bottled water that exceeded national guidelines for lead, chloride, and dissolved solids.

Unlike tap water, bottled water may also contain trace amounts of polyethylene terephthalate, antimony, bisphenol A, and other chemicals that leach from plastic bottles into water. These chemicals are linked to hormone disruption and adverse effects on the reproductive system. Although recalls of bottled water for health reasons are rare, one brand of bottled water in the U.S. experienced a major recall in 2007 because of high levels of arsenic.

In addition to these concerns, there are concerns about the high environmental cost of bottled water—from the energy and pollution caused by long-distance transportation to the manufacturing and disposal of plastic or glass bottles. Although recyclable in theory, most plastic water bottles end up in the dump. A less recognized cost of bottled water is that it undermines support for public drinking water infrastructure and treatment. If the billions spent annually on bottled water were redirected to improve drinking water infrastructure, both human health and the environment would be big winners. In Canada, tens of billions of dollars are needed to replace aging water infrastructure, while in the U.S., almost 300 billion dollars are needed.

Legitimate uses for bottled water are few

Compared to home water treatment options, bottled water is more expensive, less likely to protect your health, and worse for the environment. Legitimate uses for bottled water are few: during emergencies and humanitarian crises, in places where water is untreated or there are serious concerns about drinking water quality, and when individuals with compromised immune systems need protection. If you must purchase bottled water, avoid fancy brands from halfway across the world. Instead, buy a local brand certified by the NSF, which tests for over 160 chemical, inorganic, radiological, and microbiological contaminants and conducts annual unannounced plant inspections covering every aspect of a bottler's operation.

Contaminants of Particular Concern

The approaches mentioned so far—testing, treating, and monitoring—can all be used to avoid exposure to four common contaminants in drinking water: *Cryptosporidium*, lead, nitrates, and arsenic.

Cryptosporidium

Cryptosporidium is a microscopic parasite that lives in the intestine of infected animals and humans. It passes in the stool and has an outer shell or cyst that both allows it to survive outside the body for long periods of time and makes it resistant to chlorine-based disinfectants. It occurs mainly in lakes, streams, and rivers. In healthy adults, *Cryptosporidium* can cause minor symptoms such as diarrhea and stomach cramps, but for people with weakened immune systems, it can cause severe illness and death.

WHAT YOU CAN DO

> Boil your drinking water (see page 112). The most effective way of killing *Cryptosporidium* is to boil water for a full minute.

> Use distillation, reverse osmosis, ultraviolet light, or filtration that removes particles one micron or less in diameter. The greatest assurance of removing *Cryptosporidium* is provided by filters labeled as "absolute one micron filters" or "certified for cyst removal."

> If you have concerns about *Cryptosporidium* because a member of your household suffers from a compromised immune system, choose bottled water that has been treated using reverse osmosis, distillation, ultraviolet light, or filtration with an absolute one micron filter or smaller.

> Take the precautions described here for drinking water as well as for water used to brush teeth, make ice cubes, and wash fruits and vegetables.

BOIL WATER ADVISORIES «

Boil water advisories are public health announcements directing people to boil their tap water for drinking, washing fruits and vegetables, brushing teeth, or preparing food, beverages, and ice cubes. Severely immunocompromised individuals should always boil their tap water for these purposes (or use certified bottled water). It is not necessary to boil tap water for other household purposes, such as showering, doing laundry, or washing dishes.

Boil water advisories are issued when there is evidence that a water supply is, or may be, contaminated with dangerous levels of bacteria, viruses, or parasites, or when the water is cloudy (high turbidity can mask the presence of pathogens). Some boil water advisories are issued on a precautionary basis, such as when the local water distribution system undergoes emergency repairs. Even if you have a home water treatment system, you should still follow boil water advisories.

To boil water in a way that kills all disease-causing organisms, bring it to a rolling boil for one minute. Pour the cooled water into a clean container and refrigerate it until needed. At elevations over 2,000 meters (6,560 feet) water boils at a lower temperature and will need to be boiled for at least two minutes to kill all disease-causing organisms.

When out in the wild, disinfect all untreated drinking water—even if it looks clean—by boiling it for one minute (two minutes at higher elevations) or by passing it through a filter with an absolute pore size of 0.1 micron or smaller and adding a chemical disinfectant.

Lead

Public water suppliers regularly test for lead. However, these tests are conducted on the water as it leaves the treatment facility rather than when it comes out of your tap. Lead from corroding pipes, solder, fixtures, faucets, and fittings can enter your water as it travels through the distribution system or the plumbing in your home. The amount of lead in your water depends on the types and quantities of minerals in the water, how long the water stays in the pipes, the amount of wear in the pipes, and the acidity and temperature of the water. Homes built before 1950 often have lead distribution lines and service connections, while homes built before 1986 may have lead in their plumbing systems. Recent tests in Washington, D.C., found that one in ten homes had lead in tap water at up to five times the Environmental Protection Agency's standards. Similar tests in older homes in Toronto found more than half had lead levels above the acceptable level. If you are concerned about the possibility of lead in your drinking water, it's best to test.

> **Homes built before 1950 often have lead distribution lines and service connections, while homes built before 1986 may have lead in their plumbing systems**

WHAT YOU CAN DO

> Remove any lead from your household plumbing and advocate for its removal from your water supplier's distribution system.

> Install a home water treatment system that uses an activated carbon filter, reverse osmosis, or distillation to remove lead. For best results, the system should be installed on all taps that are used for drinking water and be certified for the removal of lead by the NSF, Underwriters Laboratories (www.UL.com), or the Water Quality Association (www.wqa.org).

> Do not boil water in an attempt to get rid of lead—boiling will actually increase lead concentrations.

> Always use water from the cold tap rather than the hot tap for drinking, boiling, cooking, and mixing infant formula. Lead dissolves more easily in hot water.

> Until you address the source of the lead in your water, do not drink the first water to come out of your tap, especially in the morning when the water has been in contact with the pipes overnight. Instead, flush your system by running the tap for several minutes and save this water for another use, such as watering houseplants.

Nitrates

One of every ten American households that rely on private wells faces nitrate levels that exceed the maximum level recommended by government. Water is contaminated with nitrates from agricultural fertilizers, livestock manure, or septic tank effluent. The main concern with nitrate contamination is blue baby syndrome (methemoglobinemia), which can lower IQ or be fatal without immediate medical attention. Infants most at risk for blue baby syndrome are those who are very young or already sick when they consume food, water, or formula that is high in nitrates. Consumption of drinking water contaminated by nitrates can also cause miscarriages.

WHAT YOU CAN DO

> If you live in an agricultural area and drink water from a well, test your water annually.

> Avoid using water high in nitrates for drinking. This is especially important for infants and young children, nursing mothers, pregnant women, and elderly people.

> Do not boil your water in an attempt to reduce nitrate levels—boiling will actually increase nitrate concentrations.

Arsenic

Over a lifetime, consuming water that contains high levels of arsenic can increase the risk of skin cancer and cancer of the bladder, liver, kidneys, and lungs. While utility companies are required by law to keep arsenic levels in drinking water below 10 parts per billion (7 ppb in Australia), no safeguards exist for people who quench their thirst with water from private wells. An inexpensive lab test can determine whether a well is contaminated with arsenic. High levels of arsenic have been found in drinking water in regions of the U.S., Australia, and Canada.

WHAT YOU CAN DO

> If you live in an area where arsenic may be a problem, have your water tested. The U.S. Geological Survey offers maps of arsenic levels at http://water.usgs.gov/nawqa/trace/arsenic/.

> Water treatment systems using reverse osmosis and distillation can reduce arsenic levels; water softeners and pitcher filters cannot.

> Call on governments to strengthen existing drinking water standards for arsenic to provide more protection from the risk of cancer.

Act to Protect Water Supplies

Remedial action will be needed less often if we reduce the number of contaminants entering local ecosystems. Regardless of where your water comes from, it is important to protect water bodies from pollution:

> Do not dispose of household cleaners, used oil, unused medications, or other hazardous waste products down toilets or drains. Never dispose of hazardous waste in ditches, rivers, lakes, or wooded areas.

> If you live near a surface water supply and have a septic system, make sure your septic system is in good operating condition. Failing septic systems are one of the major sources of nitrates in surface water. Never dispose of human waste where it can enter water supplies.

> When fueling watercraft or other vehicles, take care not to spill gasoline or oil into lakes or rivers.

Advice for Parents

Several of the contaminants discussed in this chapter, including lead and nitrates, pose a particular threat to babies and young children and can cause lifelong problems. Protect your children's health by taking the following steps:

> If you live in an older home or an older neighborhood, have your water tested for lead. If tests reveal elevated lead levels, either remove the source (by replacing pipes that contain lead) or use a home water treatment system that is certified to remove lead.

> If you live on a farm or near an agricultural community, have your water tested for nitrates. If tests reveal elevated levels, ensure that infants and young children are provided with water from a safe, alternate source. Pregnant women and nursing mothers should also avoid foods and beverages made with water high in nitrates.

> Remember that boiling water will not reduce lead or nitrate levels but will actually make matters worse by concentrating these substances.

Wrap-up

If you rely on a small public water system or a private source of water, then you need to be more proactive in evaluating the safety of your drinking water. The presence of *Cryptosporidium*, *E. coli* O157:H7, nitrates, and arsenic in your drinking water may threaten your health. If you rely on a larger public water system, contaminants of significant concern include lead and disinfection by-products. The water at schools, daycare centers, nursing homes, offices, and other locations is subject to the same contamination problems as the water at your home.

Experts agree that we need to address threats to water quality all the way from sources to taps. The key elements of a comprehensive approach are protection of water sources (to keep raw water as clean as possible), adequate treatment (including disinfection, filtration, and additional processes to remove or inactivate contaminants), a well-maintained distribution system, strong water quality standards, and rigorous enforcement. A comprehensive approach also includes regular inspection, testing, monitoring, and operator training and certification; public notice procedures, reporting, and involvement; contingency planning, research, and adequate funding.

Drink Safe Water

> Find out what, if any, contaminants are in your tap water.

> Determine whether levels of contaminants in your tap water pose a health risk.

> If necessary, select a home water treatment system that meets your needs, and install and maintain the system according to the manufacturer's instructions.

> Use NSF-certified bottled water in place of tap water only when absolutely necessary—during an emergency or a boil water advisory, and to protect a household member with a compromised immune system.

> Protect water supplies by keeping hazardous substances and human waste out of rivers, streams, and lakes.

6 THE THINGS WE BUY AND USE

The answer to the age-old philosophical question: why are we here? Plastic.

George Carlin

WHEN WE BREATHE, eat, or drink, it's obvious that whatever chemicals are in the air, food, and water will enter our nose or mouth en route to our lungs or stomach. However, when we come in contact with a vast array of consumer products—furniture, electronic goods, clothing, frying pans, toys, kitchen cleaners, and plastic food containers—few of us imagine that chemicals from these items will somehow end up in our bodies. And yet they do. Through the conventional routes of exposure—inhalation, consumption, and contact—these chemicals insidiously become part of us. What we put in the environment, we put in ourselves. Every person living in the western world has a body burden that probably includes flame retardants, stain repellents, phthalates, heavy metals, pesticides, and hundreds of other unwelcome chemicals originating in the things we buy.

There is a widespread belief that if you can buy something from a store, then government regulators have determined it is safe to use. This is a false assumption. Ordinary consumer products contain ingredients that can cause cancer, impair normal brain development in children, disrupt the vital functions of our hormone systems, and damage our reproductive systems. There has been a rise in some kinds of birth defects that scientists are concerned may be related to environmental chemical exposures. For example, there has been a doubling of hypospadias, a condition in which the opening of the penis is located on the underside rather than the tip. Almost one in one hundred males in the U.S. are now born with this condition (which usually requires surgical correction).

The degree of regulatory oversight of chemicals and consumer products around the world is nowhere near sufficient to ensure that people's health is protected

The degree of regulatory oversight of chemicals and consumer products around the world is nowhere near sufficient to ensure that people's health is protected. Arsenic, asbestos, barium, cadmium, lead, mercury, and gamma-hydroxybutyrate (known as the date rape drug) have been found recently in children's toys imported from China.

Governments are just now engaging in the arduous process of evaluating tens of thousands of chemicals used by industry for decades. Canada has identified roughly four thousand chemicals of concern from a list of more than twenty-three thousand. Those four thousand are now subject to closer scrutiny as the government struggles to decide how best to protect people from harm. In many cases, there is little scientific research on how these chemicals affect human health. In the U.S., the situation is even worse. The Toxic Substances Control Act was passed in 1976, but of the sixty-two thousand chemicals in commerce at that time, the U.S. Environmental Protection Agency has required extensive testing of only two hundred, and banned a grand total of five substances or groups of substances (PCBs, CFCs, dioxins, asbestos, and hexavalent chromium). Even for the three thousand high-production-volume chemicals (produced or imported at levels exceeding 450,000 kilograms or 1,000,000 pounds per year), basic toxicity data are lacking for 93%. The results of this reckless disregard are sometimes difficult to believe. For example, some plywood imported from China and sold in the U.S. contains levels of formaldehyde, a known carcinogen, so high that the product could not be sold legally in Japan, Europe, or, ironically, China.

Are the risks worth it? Do we really need toxic carpet cleaners, nail polish removers, nonstick cookware, and fabric brighteners? Or would our lives be simpler and safer without some of the products that advertisers seduce us into buying? While it is daunting to learn that thousands of potentially harmful chemicals are used in millions of everyday consumer products, there are steps you can take to reduce or eliminate your exposure to these hazards.

Given the countless different products available in stores and online—a typical Walmart carries more than a million—it helps to focus on six groups of products and seven specific substances that pose serious threats to human health and the environment. The six groups of products are pesticides, cosmetics and personal care products, household cleaning products, antibacterial products, nanotechnology products, and medications. The seven substances are lead, mercury, polyvinyl chloride, phthalates, bisphenol A, polybrominated diphenyl ethers, and perfluorinated chemicals. Although the complete extent of the health threats posed by some of these products and substances is not yet known, there is enough evidence to be concerned and take steps to reduce your risk. Minimizing your exposure is especially important if you are pregnant or planning to become pregnant, have young children, or suffer from chemical sensitivities. Products that are inherently dangerous but are used by choice—tobacco, alcohol, and other drugs—will not be addressed here. If you are hooked on any of these addictive substances, then you have bigger health problems to worry about than the environmental hazards discussed in this book, and addressing these should be your first priority.

Minimizing your exposure is especially important if you are pregnant or planning to become pregnant, have young children, or suffer from chemical sensitivities

Consumer Products

Both short-term exposure and long-term exposure to hazardous consumer products pose health threats. Short-term exposures, mainly accidental, result in poisonings, which can involve acute adverse effects ranging from headaches and nausea to respiratory failure and death. Over 2.5 million Americans and Canadians are poisoned every year by products commonly found in homes, including medications, cosmetics, cleaning products, and pesticides. Long-term exposures may contribute to other kinds of health effects, including cancer, respiratory disease, neurological diseases such as Alzheimer's and Parkinson's, and damage to the reproductive system.

Over 2.5 million Americans and Canadians are poisoned every year by products commonly found in homes

Before considering specific ways to reduce your exposure to hazardous substances in consumer products, go to the root of the problem: Buy less stuff! As far as advice goes, this gem has many virtues. It's simple, easy to remember, and guaranteed to save money, free up more of your time, and reduce stress. As a result of these other benefits, buying less stuff will probably make you happier. It will also alleviate some of the pressure on our beleaguered planet, since products that harm humans generally have deleterious effects on other species and the environment.

Pesticides
Pesticide is a catch-all term for chemicals engineered to kill insects, weeds, fungi, and rodents. Common pesticides used in many households include mothballs, weed-and-feed lawn products, ant baits, flea repellents, and bug sprays. Pressure-treated lumber, often used for building decks, playgrounds, and other backyard structures, used to be impregnated with a pesticide containing arsenic, chromium, and copper. Although sales of this type of pressure-treated lumber were phased out in 2005, millions of homes still have decks and other structures that contain arsenic, which can leach from the wood and contaminate soil and water.

Pesticides poison more than one hundred thousand people a year in the U.S. and Canada, including more than fifty-five thousand children under the age of six. Most of these avoidable poisonings occur because pesticides are lying around the home, garage, or yard, improperly stored. Prolonged and repeated pesticide exposure is linked to long-term health problems, including damage to the reproductive system, cancer, neurological diseases, developmental deficits, and birth defects. Three-quarters of American households continue to use these dangerous chemicals.

WHAT YOU CAN DO

> Avoid using pesticides in and around your home. There are almost always safer alternatives, including effective nonchemical methods of pest control. Prevention is the best approach. For example, prevent problems with ants and termites by sealing access points with caulking or similar material and not allowing wooden building materials to come in direct contact with soil. Keep your home clean. Store foods, especially sugary ones, in secure glass or metal containers. Wash pets and indoor plants frequently.

> If, despite the risks, you do choose to use pesticides, find the least toxic product available. For example, borax is effective against ants but generally not toxic to people. If you hire a professional pest management company, choose one with a good reputation and make your concerns about toxic chemicals known. If you apply pesticides yourself, read the label and follow the directions; never use more than the recommended amount; and wear proper protective clothing. Never use pesticides or have them applied by professionals when children or pregnant women are nearby.

> Do not use mothballs. Naphthalene and paradichlorobenzene can irritate lungs and are linked to cancer and reproductive problems.

> Store pesticides in a secure locked location that is inaccessible to young children.

> Keep pesticides in their original containers to prevent confusion and misidentification, and to maintain access to the instructions for minimizing risks.

> Dispose of unwanted pesticides safely. Check with your local hazardous household waste facility, recycling center, or poison control center for advice on safe disposal. Never put pesticides in the garbage, pour them down the drain, or flush them down the toilet.

> Keep the number for your local poison control center near the phone.

> If your home has a deck, playground, or other structure built with pressure-treated lumber purchased before 2005, you need to take action. Your best approach is to seal the wood with an oil-based, semi-transparent stain on a regular basis (every one or two years). Replace any pressure-treated lumber in direct contact with soil or compost being used in a garden for growing food. Remove contaminated soil from underneath any pressure-treated structures or create barriers to prevent access by children and pets. Dispose of treated lumber through your community's hazardous waste program—never burn this kind of wood (you'll create highly toxic smoke and ash) and never use it for mulch or compost.

> Follow the excellent advice on organic gardening available at www.organicgardening.com.

> Advocate for a ban on cosmetic pesticide use in your community. Two Canadian provinces and more than 150 Canadian municipalities have passed laws prohibiting the use of pesticides for cosmetic purposes. In Quebec, where this approach was pioneered, the proportion of households using pesticides quickly dropped by 50% and in some communities cosmetic pesticide use plummeted by 90%.

Cosmetics and Personal Care Products

Each day the average person slathers on nine personal care products that can contain more than 120 different chemicals, including toluene, formaldehyde, dibutyl phthalate (DBP), 1,4-dioxane, parabens, phenyl-enediamine, sodium lauryl sulfate (SLS), and fragrances. Although the concentrations of these chemicals are generally low, their effects on health can be significant. Toluene is a developmental neurotoxin, meaning it harms the brains of fetuses, babies, and young children. It can also affect the central nervous system, causing headaches, dizziness, and fatigue. Formaldehyde causes cancer and irritates the eyes, nose, skin, and throat. DBP is an endocrine-disrupting chemical implicated in the feminization of baby boys. The cancer-causing 1,4-dioxane is an impurity rather than an ingredient found in shampoos, soaps, bubble bath, and other personal care products—so 1,4-dioxane never appears on product labels. Parabens are used as preservatives in a wide variety of personal care products and have been linked to breast cancer and damaged sperm. On labels you'll see them identified by type—ethylparaben, methylparaben, butylparaben, propylparaben, and isobutylparaben are common. Phenylenediamine is used in hair dyes and can irritate the lungs, cause severe allergic reactions, and harm the nervous system. SLS was initially used as an industrial degreaser and garage floor cleaner. Now it is used in soaps, shampoos, dish detergents, and toothpaste. Fragrance is code for a range of chemicals (often including phthalates); some can cause serious allergic reactions.

More than a thousand companies have agreed to abide by the strict health protection principles established by the global Campaign for Safe Cosmetics

There is good news on the cosmetics front. Europe has banned the use of more than thirteen hundred substances in cosmetics because they are known or suspected of causing cancer, genetic changes, birth defects, or damage to the reproductive system. In Europe, Canada, and the U.S., progress has been made in requiring companies to disclose ingredients, although more work needs to be done to make this information comprehensible to the average person. Canada recently created a Cosmetic Ingredient Hotlist that prohibits or restricts the use of hundreds of chemicals and contaminants such as hydroquinone, selenium, nitrosamines, and 1,4-dioxane—all of which the U.S. still allows. More than a thousand companies have agreed to abide by the strict health protection principles established by the global Campaign for Safe Cosmetics (www.safecosmetics.org). The agreement requires companies to remove toxic chemicals from their products, replace them with safer alternatives, and meet more stringent European rules.

WHAT YOU CAN DO

> Avoid personal care products containing lead, mercury, placenta, phthalates, petroleum by-products, nanoparticles, parabens, diethanolamine, triethanolamine, glycol ethers, toluene, and sodium lauryl sulfate. A helpful database containing information on more than forty thousand products is available at www.cosmeticsdatabase.com/special/whatnottobuy/.

> Avoid shampoo, bubble bath, and other products that list polyethylene glycol, ethoxylated surfactants, or foaming agents on the label.

> Pregnant women (and women attempting to become pregnant) should limit the use of cosmetics and personal care products, as some toxic substances can be passed on to the developing fetus. Particular products to avoid are perfumes, hair spray, body lotion, and deodorant.

> Use products labeled "fragrance-free" or "perfume-free." Avoid products described as "unscented," since these may merely use other chemicals to mask odors or to dull the sense of smell.

> Read labels skeptically. Choose products with fewer ingredients, and ingredients that you can identify. Be wary of products described as "natural" or "organic." Although organic food is regulated, these terms have no legal meaning in the world of cosmetics and personal care products.

> Avoid the use of powders and sprays, as these are more easily inhaled and can get into your eyes.

Household Cleaning Products
Household cleaning products are involved in more than 200,000 poisoning incidents each year in the U.S. and Canada, with more than half of these poisonings harming children age five or younger. Chemicals

commonly found in household cleaning products can trigger asthma attacks, harm the reproductive system, and cause developmental difficulties. Particularly problematic products include drain cleaners, spot removers, carpet cleaners, oven cleaners, glass cleaners, tub-tile-and-shower cleaners, toilet bowl cleaners, metal cleaners and polishes, pool chemicals, and furniture polish. Bleach and ammonia, two common cleaners, are also highly hazardous. Worse yet, if mixed, ammonia and bleach react by forming chlorine gas and chloramines that can cause permanent damage to the lungs.

WHAT YOU CAN DO

> Make your own cleaning products from nontoxic ingredients (see page 128). Hot water and soap are often sufficient.

> Choose from the many eco-friendly commercial cleaning products available today. Dr. Bronner's, Seventh Generation, Nature Clean, Ecover, Earth Friendly Products, and Simply Clean make all-purpose cleaners, laundry products, and cleaners for floors, kitchens, and bathrooms.

> Use a plunger or a plumber's snake to unplug toilets and drains.

> Choose products that pour instead of those that spray to minimize the risk of inhaling these substances or getting them in your eyes.

> Read labels carefully and avoid products that say Danger, Poison, Warning, Corrosive, Explosive, or Flammable.

> Look for carpet cleaners and spot removers that do not contain TCE (trichloroethylene) and PERC (perchloroethylene). Both are carcinogens.

> Never mix bleach and ammonia or products containing these substances.

> Store cleaning products in a locked cupboard that is inaccessible to young children.

> Keep products in their original containers to avoid misidentification.

> Dispose of unwanted products in a safe manner.

ALTERNATIVES TO COMMON
HOUSEHOLD CLEANERS

DRAIN CLEANER. Use half a cup of baking soda, then half a cup of white vinegar followed by several cups of boiling water.

GLASS CLEANER. Mix 15 milliliters (1 tablespoon) of vinegar or lemon juice in 1 liter (1 quart) of water. Spray on and use newspaper or old rags to wipe dry.

TOILET BOWL CLEANER. Use a toilet brush and baking soda or vinegar. This will clean but not disinfect.

DISINFECTANT. Use hydrogen peroxide, a safer disinfectant than chlorine bleach.

FURNITURE POLISH. Mix 5 milliliters (1 teaspoon) of lemon juice in 0.5 liter (1 pint) of mineral or vegetable oil, and wipe furniture.

CARPET DEODORIZER. Sprinkle dry carpets liberally with baking soda, brush in gently, wait at least fifteen minutes and vacuum. Repeat if necessary.

PLANT SPRAYS. Wipe leaves with mild soap and water; rinse.

Antibacterial Products

Germ-killing consumer products are flooding the market in response to fears about killer bacteria, new viruses, and dramatic disease outbreaks. Everything from hand soap and facial tissues to socks and underwear is being promoted for killing germs and, by implication, protecting your health. In fact, experts worry that these products could have the opposite effect. First, let's distinguish this new wave of consumer products from conventional disinfectants such as bleach and hydrogen peroxide. Disinfectants are useful for killing a range of bacteria and viruses found in bathrooms and kitchens. Most of the new generation of germ-killing products rely on triclosan, a chemical that kills bacteria but has no effect on viruses—meaning it is useless against common illnesses such as colds and flu. Antibacterials are useful in hospitals and other medical settings where people are particularly vulnerable, but they have no proven utility in the average home.

Unfortunately, triclosan is structurally similar to PCBs and dioxins, both highly toxic substances. Triclosan bioaccumulates in fish and has been detected in human breast milk, as well as the urine of three in four Americans. Researchers have discovered that exposure to triclosan at low levels, similar to those found today in many North American streams and rivers, can disrupt the normal development of frogs. Scientists also worry that the widespread use of triclosan and similar antibacterials could contribute to the growth of superbugs—bacteria that are resistant to chemicals.

WHAT YOU CAN DO

> Avoid antibacterial consumer products. Ordinary soap does a perfectly good job of cleaning, without posing an unnecessary risk to human health and the environment.

> Wash hands often with soap and hot water, especially after going to the bathroom and before cooking or eating.

> Keep kitchens and bathrooms clean.

Nanotechnology Products

Nanotechnology is a rapidly growing field that involves manufacturing and using material at a scale of less than 100 nanometers. A nanometer is one-billionth of a meter. To put this in perspective, an average sheet of paper is 100,000 nanometers thick. Proponents of nanotechnology have visions of ultramicroscopic cameras that flow through your bloodstream to identify constrictions or blockages, bulletproof clothing the thickness of spandex, and supercomputers the size of a grain of salt. Although nanotechnology sounds like something straight out of science fiction, nanotech products are already on store shelves. For example, nanoparticles of titanium dioxide and zinc oxide are used in sunscreen and toothpaste.

Although nanotechnology sounds like something straight out of science fiction, nanotech products are already on store shelves

Nanotechnology offers tremendous promise, but some applications have the potential to harm human health. Although there is still a dearth of knowledge about the possible adverse effects of nanotechnology, early toxicological studies raise serious concerns. Nanoparticles can be inhaled, ingested, or absorbed through the skin. Once inside the body, nanoparticles can enter the blood system, be transported to the spleen, liver, kidneys, and heart, and can penetrate the blood-brain barrier. Scientists have observed genetic damage, respiratory illness, cardiovascular disease, and cancer in laboratory animals exposed to nanoparticles. In a disturbing display of our inability to learn from the mistakes of the past (think CFCs or PCBs), there is little or no regulatory oversight of nanotech products anywhere in the world, and no requirement that the presence of nanoparticles be indicated on product labels.

WHAT YOU CAN DO

> Avoid cosmetic products and foods that contain nanoparticles. For cosmetics that do not contain nanoparticles, see www.cosmeticsdatabase.com/index.php. Also avoid consumer

products such as socks and underwear that contain silver nanoparticles, as scientists are concerned that these will tend to exacerbate antibiotic resistance and may wash off, causing environmental damage in water bodies.

> Urge governments to require both extensive safety testing and clear labeling of nanotechnology products.

> Learn more about nanotechnology. The Woodrow Wilson International Center for Scholars has an informative website (www.nanotechproject. org).

Medications

Both prescription and over-the-counter drugs can be toxic. As prescription drug use increases, so do concerns about the effect of discarded pharmaceutical products on ecosystems and human health. Studies show that almost half of North American households dispose of unused or expired medications by putting them in the garbage, flushing them down the toilet, or pouring them down the drain. This poses a threat to fish, wildlife, and humans, who may be exposed through the accumulation of drugs in drinking water.

WHAT YOU CAN DO

> Do not throw out medications of any kind—pills, liquids, or ointments—by putting them into the garbage, flushing them down the toilet, or pouring them down the drain. Instead, return them to your local pharmacist, who will dispose of them safely.

> Store all medication in a locked cupboard that is inaccessible to young children.

> Follow instructions on the label carefully.

Hazardous Substances

Many substances used to manufacture goods are toxic. As a result, the first signs of a threat to human health often come from work settings where people are exposed to higher concentrations of specific toxic substances over extended periods. In some cases, subsequent research reveals that consumers are also vulnerable. A recent example is diacetyl, a chemical used to provide artificial butter flavor in microwave popcorn and other processed foods. In 2000, epidemiologists discovered that workers in factories where microwave popcorn was being manufactured suffered from high rates of a devastating and sometimes fatal respiratory illness called bronchiolitis obliterans, or popcorn lung. In 2007, the first case of a consumer suffering from bronchiolitis obliterans as a result of heavy microwave popcorn consumption was reported.

Seven hazardous substances commonly found in a wide array of consumer products are lead, mercury, polyvinyl chloride, phthalates, bisphenol A, polybrominated diphenyl ethers, and perfluorinated chemicals. Although these heavy metals and chemicals can be found in all kinds of different products, their presence will rarely be reported on labels or accompanying product information.

Lead

It is well known that young children exposed to lead can suffer from decreased bone and muscle growth, poor coordination, impaired hearing, behavioral problems, damage to the nervous system and kidneys, developmental delays, and reduced intelligence. New research links childhood lead exposure to smaller brain size and violent criminal behavior. For children, there is no safe level of exposure. Lead poses a threat to adults too, especially menopausal women and the elderly. As bones thin with age, lead is released into the blood, potentially contributing to cataracts, Alzheimer's disease, Parkinson's disease, high blood pressure, cardiovascular disease, and impaired kidney function. Lead exposure also increases the risk of heart disease and stroke. In one major study, adults with elevated blood lead levels were found to be 2.5 times more likely than adults with lower levels to die of a stroke, 89% more likely to die of a heart attack, and 55% more likely to die of cardiovascular diseases.

Although no longer added to gasoline or paint, lead continues to pose a threat in consumer products, including toys, crystal glassware, costume jewelry, hair dyes, mini-blinds, and makeup. In 2006, an American child died after swallowing a heart-shaped charm from a bracelet included as a gift with the purchase of new shoes. Subsequent tests determined that the charm was 99.1% lead. In the recent wave of unsafe products from China, many toys, infant bibs, and children's lunch boxes were contaminated with high concentrations of lead. Lead-based paint was banned decades ago but remains in about 24 million American housing units and over 3 million Australian homes. One in four Canadian children under the age of five lives in an older home where lead paint may pose an ongoing threat.

For children, there is no safe level of exposure to lead

WHAT YOU CAN DO

> If you live in an older home (built before 1978) and paint is flaking, peeling, and cracking, or if you are considering renovations, have paint tested for lead content. Pay close attention to windowsills, which are exposed to the elements and subject to wear and tear. Any activity that creates fine debris—sanding or scraping—can dramatically increase the levels of lead in a home. Consider hiring a certified lead abatement contractor to remove lead paint (in the U.S. call 1-800-424-LEAD). Do not use belt sanders, propane torches, heat guns, dry scrapers, or sandpaper because they could create lead dust and fumes. Lead-based paint that is in good condition is usually not a hazard.

> Eat meals rich in calcium, iron, and vitamin C to help block the absorption and storage of lead in your body.

> Do not store food or drinks in lead crystal glassware or imported pottery.

> Stay up-to-date on recalls of lead-contaminated products. The U.S. Consumer Product Safety Commission (www.cpsc.gov) issues recalls of products that could potentially expose children to lead. Health Canada (www.healthycanadians.gc.ca) and Australia (www.recalls.gov.au) provide a similar service.

> Test your drinking water for lead (see Chapter 5).

> Consider having your children's blood lead levels tested at age one and two if they have lived in or regularly visited homes built before 1950 with peeling paint or that had renovations completed within the past six months; have a sibling, housemate, or playmate being treated for lead poisoning; live with an adult who is exposed to lead at work or through hobby activities; or live near lead industries (e.g., lead smelter, battery-recycling plant) or a busy highway.

> Locate vegetable gardens away from older buildings to avoid using soil contaminated by lead paint. If you live near a major road, test soil for lead before establishing a vegetable garden or build raised beds and purchase soil.

Mercury

The main source of mercury exposure for most people is through the consumption of fish (see Chapter 4). However, you can also be exposed to mercury from household items that break, such as fluorescent lights, thermostats, thermometers, and barometers.

WHAT YOU CAN DO

> If you experience a small mercury spill, never try to vacuum or sweep up the mercury with a broom, as this will actually disperse it through the air where you might inhale it. Instead, follow the detailed procedure recommended by Canada's National Collaborating Centre for Environmental Health at www.ncceh.ca/files/Mercury_Spills_Nov_2007.pdf.

> Properly dispose of items that contain mercury. Never put mercury down a sink or toilet. Fluorescent lights can be recycled and other products containing mercury can be taken to hazardous waste drop-off sites.

> Buy mercury-free or low-mercury products. For example, new digital thermometers do not use mercury. There are low-mercury fluorescent light bulbs available.

> Ask your dentist for an alternative to fillings that contain mercury.

Polyvinyl Chloride

Polyvinyl chloride (also known as PVC or vinyl) is one of the most common types of plastic in the world. In fact, you may be surprised how challenging it can be to avoid PVC: it is used in everything from shower curtains and vinyl flooring to water pipes and lunch boxes. Two of the main ingredients in PVC—ethylene dichloride and vinyl chloride monomer—are known carcinogens. By-products of PVC production and disposal include dioxins, furans, PCBs, and hexachlorobenzene—all extremely toxic substances. Phthalates and heavy metals are added to PVC in the manufacturing process. According to Dr. Joe Thornton, an expert in the field of environmental impacts on health, "PVC is one of the most environmentally hazardous consumer materials ever produced." The chemicals produced and released in the manufacture of PVC cause cancer, disrupt the hormone system, impair normal child development, suppress the immune system, and lead to birth defects and brain damage.

PVC is one of the most environmentally hazardous consumer materials ever produced

WHAT YOU CAN DO

> Do not buy products made of PVC or vinyl. This includes toys, vinyl flooring, vinyl siding, vinyl shower curtains, and imitation leather goods such as vinyl bags. Look for products labeled PVC-free or vinyl-free and avoid all plastics with the number 3 in the recycling triangle or the letters PVC or V underneath the recycling symbol.

> Mention to retailers that you'd like to see PVC-free alternatives, and ask them to pass the word on to their distributors. Substitutes will eventually become easier to find.

> Encourage your church, school, local government, or company to pass a toxin-free purchasing policy that phases out the purchase of extremely toxic chemicals and products such as PVC. Links to such policies can be found at www.besafenet.com/pvc/about.htm.

Phthalates

Phthalates are chemicals widely used to soften plastics and can be found in toys, food packaging, vinyl products, teething rings, and toothbrushes. They are also used to prolong the effect of fragrances and are found in cosmetics, air fresheners, fabric softeners, and cleaning products. Lab tests on seventy-two name-brand beauty products revealed phthalates in nearly three-quarters of the products, even though these chemicals were not listed on any of the labels. Most people carry multiple kinds of phthalates in their bodies because of exposure to consumer products. Phthalates are, quite literally, everywhere. Even deep-sea jellyfish in the North Atlantic are contaminated. Phthalates migrate out of plastics and find their way into our air, food, and water. Swedish research has linked phthalates in house dust to elevated levels of asthma in children.

Phthalate exposure is both higher and more common than previously suspected, with the highest levels reported in children and women of child-bearing age. Animal tests indicate that phthalates disrupt the normal functioning of the hormone system, causing reproductive and developmental harm. Recent human studies suggest that phthalate exposures in pregnant women may lead to genital abnormalities in baby boys. The changes occurred at phthalate levels that have been measured in about one-quarter of women in the United States. Phthalates are also associated with infertility, poor sperm quality, and testicular cancer.

The European Union banned the use of six phthalates in toys and other products intended for children in 1999. California followed with a similar law in 2008 and a law covering all of the U.S. came into effect early in 2009. These laws should reduce the risk to children, although myriad other consumer products continue to contain phthalates. In contrast, Canada employed a voluntary restriction on phthalates beginning in 1998, an industry-friendly policy that was a dismal failure. A 2008 Health Canada study of seventy-two toys made of PVC found fifty-four contained phthalates. In 2009, Canada finally proposed regulations similar to those already in force in the U.S. and Europe.

WHAT YOU CAN DO

> Do not buy products made of PVC. As well as being toxic in their own right, vinyl products are likely to contain phthalates.

> Never microwave food in plastic containers. Use microwave-safe glass or ceramic containers.

> Avoid bottled water. Use a stainless steel mug or thermos or a glass jar.

> Use glass baby bottles or baby bottles made from plastic numbered 1, 2, or 5.

> Use personal care products, detergents, cleansers, and other products that do not include "fragrance" in the ingredient list because fragrances often contain phthalates. This is particularly important if you are pregnant or raising young children. Tests for phthalate in the urine of infants show that what goes on a baby—lotion, powder, shampoo—also goes in the baby. To find phthalate-free cosmetics, check the database provided by the Environmental Working Group (www.cosmeticdatabase.com).

> Do not use plug-in or fragrance-based air fresheners. Nontoxic products are available that absorb undesirable odors.

Bisphenol A

Bisphenol A (also known as BPA) is a widely used chemical found in polycarbonate plastic products, linings for food and drink cans, and sealants in dentistry. Researchers at the U.S. Centers for Disease Control and

Prevention recently detected BPA in 95% of Americans tested. Bisphenol A is linked to cancer, birth defects, cardiovascular disease, diabetes, miscarriages, impaired brain functions, and damage to reproductive systems. Recent studies indicate BPA also reduces the effectiveness of chemotherapy for cancer patients. Animal studies of low-level exposure to BPA showed stimulation of cancer cells, changes in hormones, decreased immune system function, genetic damage, decreased sperm production, and behavioral changes, including hyperactivity and increased aggressiveness. Most peer-reviewed studies conducted by independent researchers conclude that BPA is toxic at extremely low levels of exposure. Industry-funded studies reach the opposite conclusion.

There are no government safety standards limiting the amount of BPA in canned food

Independent laboratory tests in the U.S. found BPA in over half of ninety-seven cans of name-brand fruits, vegetables, soft drinks, and other common canned goods. Of all foods tested, chicken soup, infant formula, and ravioli had the highest BPA levels. Bisphenol A was found at elevated levels in one of every ten servings of canned foods and one of every three cans of infant formula. There are no government safety standards limiting the amount of BPA in canned food. Canada recently made headlines by becoming the first nation in the world to prohibit the use of bisphenol A in baby bottles.

WHAT YOU CAN DO

> Avoid polycarbonate plastic labeled 7(PC), which is used in hard plastic baby bottles, water cooler bottles, hard plastic water bottles, and plastic cutlery. Safer alternatives include glass, ceramic, stainless steel, or polypropylene. Plastics with the recycling numbers 1, 2, 4, and 5 do not contain BPA. Bio-based plastics made from corn and other crops are preferable to conventional plastics made from petroleum, but may also be labeled 7, without the PC designation. For baby bottles, sippy cups, and other products that do not contain BPA see www.zrecsguide.com.

> Never microwave food in plastic containers because the heat can cause BPA or other chemicals from the container to leach into your food. Use microwave-safe glass or ceramic containers. Avoid using plastic containers for hot food or drinks.

> Choose fresh or frozen foods over canned foods, or choose products made by companies that do not use BPA, such as Eden Organics. Of particular concern are infant formula and canned foods that are highly acidic, such as tomatoes.

> Discard old or scratched plastic bottles and sippy cups as they leach chemicals more easily and may harbor bacteria.

Polybrominated Diphenyl Ethers

Polybrominated diphenyl ethers (also known as PBDES) are a group of industrial chemicals used as flame retardants in a wide range of consumer products, including carpets, clothing, and computers. PBDES are accumulating in the environment, wildlife, and the bodies of humans at an alarming rate. In laboratory animals, exposure to tiny doses of PBDES impairs attention, learning, memory, and behavior, while exposure to higher doses has been linked to birth defects and cancer. In Canada and the U.S., exposure appears to come mainly from household dust, indoor air, and, to a lesser extent, food. The highest levels of PBDES have been detected in young children who are exposed through breast milk and through the dust on floors where they crawl and put things in their mouths.

Industry and governments in Canada, the U.S., and Australia argue that despite concerns about the effects of PBDES, current exposure levels are so low that people should not be alarmed. Still, Europe and Canada have banned most uses of PBDES, while the U.S. and Australia have brought in some weaker rules. Given the track records of industry and governments on toxic substances, it's not a bad idea to take precautions.

> Dust and vacuum regularly with a HEPA-filter vacuum, including floors, curtains, and furniture.

> Cover, replace, or dispose of any exposed polyurethane foam used in upholstered furniture, foam mattresses, car seats, and carpet padding.

> Buy computers, home electronics, clothing, bedding, and furniture from companies that have stopped using PBDEs and other brominated flame retardants. Some electronics manufacturers have publicly committed to eliminating all uses of all types of PBDEs: Acer, Apple, Dell, Eizo Nanao, HP, LG Electronics, Lenovo, Matsushita, Microsoft, Nokia, Phillips, Samsung, Sharp, Sony-Ericsson, and Toshiba. Ikea is a leader among furniture manufacturers in eliminating PBDEs from its products. H&M offers PBDE-free clothing. Wool, cotton, and hemp are naturally fire resistant. The Environmental Working Group offers helpful information on finding PBDE-free products at www.ewg.org/pbdefree.

> Although food is believed to be a minor source of exposure, you might want to eat less meat, farmed salmon, eggs, and dairy products, particularly those high in fat, where PBDEs and other toxic substances accumulate.

Perfluorinated Chemicals

Perfluorinated chemicals (also known as PFCs) are widely used in consumer products, including stain-resistant fabrics and carpets, grease-resistant packaging for fast food, stain repellents, and nonstick coatings. Many PFCs are toxic, persistent, and bioaccumulative, and are linked to cancer, liver damage, kidney damage, developmental defects, and damage to the immune system. Researchers have found a PFC called PFOA (also known as C8) in the bloodstream of 95% of the Americans they tested. A substantial proportion of PFCs detected in the bodies of Americans and Canadians come from household dust, meat, seafood, and packaged foods.

There is some progress to report in preventing health damage from PFCS. In 2002, 3M stopped using PFCS in making its Scotchgard line of products because of health and environmental concerns. In 2004, DuPont agreed to pay more than $100 million in an out-of-court settlement for contaminating water supplies in Ohio and West Virginia with PFCS. In 2005, DuPont was penalized $16 million by the U.S. Environmental Protection Agency (EPA) for failing to report information on the health risks posed by PFOA. This was the largest civil administrative penalty ever obtained by the EPA. In 2006, pressure from the EPA forced eight companies, including DuPont, to promise to reduce PFOA emissions and levels in consumer products by 95% by 2010, with complete elimination by 2015.

> A substantial proportion of PFCs detected in the bodies of Americans and Canadians come from household dust, meat, seafood, and packaged foods

WHAT YOU CAN DO
> Replace nonstick cookware and kitchen utensils with cast iron and stainless steel.

> Avoid clothing, carpeting, furniture, and other products marketed as "stain-resistant." Decline optional treatments to make products stain resistant. If the furniture you own was treated in the past, put a cover on it.

> Avoid greasy snack food and fast food that is prepared or served in coated packaging material (e.g., microwave popcorn bags, pizza boxes) since the packaging may contain PFCS. Do not store leftovers in these containers and definitely do not put these containers in the microwave.

> PFCS are added to some cosmetics (nail polish, moisturizers, and eye makeup), shaving cream, and dental floss. Avoid products listing "PTFE" or "perfluoro" in their ingredients.

Advice for Parents

Children are the most vulnerable members of society when it comes to hazardous substances in ordinary household items. The vulnerability of children relates to their physiology, behavior, and inability to protect themselves. Young children are developing rapidly, both physically and mentally, and they lack the mature detoxification mechanisms of the adult body. They also spend lots of time on the floor, like to put things in their mouths, and cannot read warning labels. More than half of all accidental poisonings in Canada and the U.S. involve children under the age of six. Exposure to lead, pesticides, mercury, and other toxic substances can inflict a terrible, and in some cases lifelong, toll on the development of children. Protect your children's health by taking the following steps:

> Green your home. Carefully evaluate the need for products that may pose a danger to your children's health. Replace hazardous products with safer substitutes. Properly dispose of unwanted materials at recycling or hazardous waste drop-off sites.

> Safely store all remaining hazardous substances, including medications, cosmetics and personal care products, cleaning products, paints, solvents, pesticides, glues, and alcohol. These items should be kept well out of reach or in a locked cabinet. Always keep hazardous substances in their original containers to prevent confusion regarding the identity of the substance or instructions for safe use.

> Check your children's toys. Even trusted brands such as Fisher Price, Mattel, and Melissa and Doug have faced product recalls. The U.S. passed a new law that came into force in 2009 placing tougher standards on toy importers and manufacturers, with a specific focus on lead and phthalates. A new consumer protection law is under development in Canada,

Exposure to lead, pesticides, mercury, and other toxic substances can inflict a terrible, and in some cases lifelong, toll on the development of children

where current rules are so weak that the government has to ask, rather than order, companies to pull hazardous products from store shelves.

> Keep an eye on recall notices issued by government. In the U.S., see www.recalls.gov; in Canada, see www.healthycanadians.gc.ca; and in Australia, see www.recalls.gov.au.

> Avoid soft plastic toys unless labeled free from PVC and phthalates.

> Check with reliable independent certification organizations (www.healthytoys.org).

> Be wary of brightly painted wooden toys and colored plastic toys unless they are made in North America, Australia, or Europe.

> Buy local.

> Be aware that if you come in contact with hazardous substances at work such as lead and asbestos you can unintentionally bring these home and expose your family to them.

> Limit use of lotions, soaps, and powders on infants.

> Take additional precautions if planning a pregnancy or while pregnant to avoid chemicals that harm the reproductive system, cause developmental problems, or are carcinogenic (see page 144).

Wrap-up

Making your home into a healthy place is well worth the time and effort. The good news is that for almost every kind of product containing hazardous substances, there are safer substitutes available. In some cases, safer products do cost more. However, the low prices of products containing dangerous chemicals do not take adverse effects on your health into account. Once this factor enters the equation, going green becomes an obvious choice. Paying a little extra to protect your health is a smart investment.

CANCER AND THE ENVIRONMENT «

ONE IN THREE people living in industrialized nations today will get cancer—partly because people are living longer, partly because other diseases have been vanquished, and partly because we live in a society where carcinogens are ubiquitous. Cancer is a disease that develops over many years and has many causes, making it difficult to say why a particular person does or does not develop cancer. Reports suggest that up to 90% of cancers are due to environmental factors rather than genetic makeup or another individual characteristic. This statistic is based on the fact that fewer than 10% of cancers can be attributed to factors unique to specific individuals, such as elevated hormone levels or weakened immune systems. However, it is important to understand that this statistic uses a very broad definition of "environmental factors."

The 90% figure includes lifestyle choices such as cigarette smoking, excessive alcohol consumption, poor diet, and lack of exercise. A significantly smaller proportion of cancer cases is caused by environmental hazards such as ultraviolet radiation, ionizing radiation, bacteria, viruses, asbestos, and chemicals such as dioxins, benzene, formaldehyde, polycyclic aromatic hydrocarbons, arsenic, beryllium, cadmium, vinyl chloride, drinking water disinfection by-products, and diesel exhaust. At least twenty chemicals used in pesticides have proven to be carcinogenic in animals, and higher rates of certain cancers are found in farmers and workers who apply pesticides on the ground or from the air. Experts are concerned that exposure to environmental contaminants is associated with increasing rates of thyroid cancer and non-Hodgkin's lymphoma in young people.

Act to minimize your risk of cancer:

> Do not use any tobacco products—cigarettes, cigars, snuff, chewing tobacco, or pipe tobacco.

> Exercise regularly, at least thirty minutes daily.

> Avoid high-calorie and high-fat foods, minimize consumption of red and preserved meats, and emphasize vegetables, fruits, and whole grains in your diet.

> Drink alcohol in moderation, if at all.

> Limit your time in the sun, especially if you are fair-skinned.

> Test your home for radon, and if levels are elevated, act to reduce them.

> Avoid pesticides in your food, home, garden, and community.

> Make sure work areas are well ventilated when using solvents and other products containing volatile organic compounds.

> Avoid exposure to diesel exhaust and other vehicle fumes.

> Do not burn garbage in your backyard.

> Have medical and dental x-rays only when absolutely necessary, and make sure the technician provides you with a shield to protect body parts not being examined.

> Be aware that cancer rates are higher in certain industries, including construction, metal working, mining, and farming. Take appropriate precautions at work to avoid exposure to hazardous substances. Ask your employer to provide Material Safety Data Sheets for any toxic chemicals that may be present in your work environment, and use personal protective equipment when necessary.

> Support groups working for cancer prevention (currently most money goes to research for cures).

> Demand that governments enact and enforce laws and policies eliminating carcinogens in air, food, water, and consumer products.

While the primary focus in this chapter is on reducing the health risks of environmental hazards, there is no doubt that making your home a cleaner, greener, safer place will pay environmental dividends as well. Our seemingly unstoppable drive for stuff has profound environmental consequences. Study after study illustrates how our ecological footprints are larger than the planet's capacity to produce sufficient resources and absorb our waste. Ironically, our myopic focus on material goods actually undermines our happiness. Research indicates that people with smaller ecological footprints lead happier lives. By buying fewer things and avoiding toxic products and goods with harmful ingredients or components, you'll reduce the size of your footprint and contribute to cleaner air, improved water quality, and healthier ecosystems and wildlife.

The low prices of products containing dangerous chemicals do not take adverse effects on your health into account

Live in a Healthy Home

> Buy less stuff and choose products with less packaging.

> Find nontoxic alternatives to pesticides.

> Use green cleaning products.

> Avoid products made with paradichlorobenzene, triclosan, lead, mercury, polyvinyl chloride, phthalates, bisphenol A, PBDEs, or PFCs.

> Use alternatives to plastic as much as possible—glass, stainless steel, cloth, and wood. Avoid plastics with the recycling numbers 3, 6, and 7 (PC). Never use plastic containers in the microwave oven.

> Keep all hazardous household products in their original containers, store them in locked locations inaccessible to children, and dispose of them in a safe manner.

> Avoid consumer products with strong or long-lasting smells.

> Stop using any products that irritate your eyes, throat, nose, or lungs.

> Avoid products with long lists of complicated, unpronounceable chemical ingredients.

> Read labels and be skeptical of certain "green" claims. Consumer Reports evaluates claims made on labels at www.greenerchoices.org/eco-labels/, and the National Institutes of Health provides information on thousands of household products at http://hpd.nlm.nih.gov/.

7 THE PHYSICAL HAZARDS WE FACE

All you have to do is go down to the bottom of your swimming pool and hold your breath.

David Miller, former U.S. Department of Energy spokesperson, on protecting yourself from nuclear radiation

WHAT DO NOISE, sunshine, and cell phone transmissions have in common? They are all physical environmental hazards—dangers that tend to be overshadowed by chemical and biological hazards.

Physical environmental hazards can pose a serious threat to human health. For example, the most dangerous item most people own is their car, truck, van, or SUV. Motor vehicle accidents kill over 100,000 people annually in the U.S., Canada, Australia, and Europe, while maiming millions more. Other physical environmental hazards include extreme temperatures (hot and cold) and radiation from nuclear power plants, power lines, and x-rays. Fortunately, there are simple steps you can take to dramatically reduce the health risks posed by physical hazards.

Motor Vehicles

The world would be a much safer place if more people chose alternatives to driving. Some of the negative effects of vehicle pollution—cancer, respiratory illness, cardiovascular disease, and adverse effects on reproduction and fetal development—were chronicled in Chapter 2. The latest data from Canada and the U.S. show that every year almost fifty thousand people die and 3 million more are injured in vehicle crashes. The annual cost of accidents is over $250 billion in the U.S. alone. More Americans have died in traffic accidents than in all the wars the U.S. has fought during its history. Based on current trends, almost every American living today has been or will be injured in a motor vehicle accident at some point in life.

More Americans have died in traffic accidents than in all the wars the U.S. has fought during its history

Globally, an estimated 1.2 million people are killed and 50 million injured annually. That's more than three thousand deaths per day! By 2020, traffic accidents are expected to be the third largest cause of global health problems. If everyone owned cars at the same rate as Americans (where cars outnumber drivers), there would be more than 5 billion cars in the world instead of fewer than 1 billion and the carnage on roads would be even worse.

WHAT YOU CAN DO

> Walk or ride a bicycle. You will burn no fossil fuels, produce no harmful emissions, save money, and gain the health benefits of exercise. Roughly half the vehicle trips a typical driver takes involve distances of less than 5 kilometers (3 miles)—trips that can easily be done by biking or walking. Perhaps the most compelling argument in favor of walking and cycling is that these modes of travel will make you happier. Many cyclists rate their journey to and from work as one of the best parts of their day whereas most drivers describe commuting as stressful and unpleasant.

> Choose public transit. Your trip will be safer, more relaxing, less costly, and far more environmentally friendly. According to the U.S. National Safety Council, buses and trains are at least twenty times safer than cars.

> Take advantage of technological advances that allow you to telecommute and use videoconferencing. Spending less time traveling for work, meetings, and presentations will make you happier and more productive.

> Join a car-sharing organization that allows you to pay for access to a vehicle when you need one. You'll not only reduce environmental impacts, you'll save money and avoid the hassles of vehicle ownership—purchasing, insuring, and repairing a car. According to recent studies, each car-sharing vehicle can replace five to twenty privately owned vehicles, leading to less traffic congestion, fewer accidents, fewer greenhouse gas emissions, and less air pollution.

> Improve your driving habits. Slowing down is the single best way to reduce both the rate and severity of accidents. Courses on defensive driving and eco-driving are widely available. Eco-driving refers to a range of actions that reduce fuel consumption, carbon dioxide emissions, air pollution, noise, vehicle repair and maintenance costs, driver and passenger stress, and accident rates.

> The greenest choice you can make is to not own a motor vehicle. However, if you must own one, buy the most fuel-efficient vehicle able to meet your needs. Hybrids, which have both gas motors and electric engines, are today's environmentally superior choice. Fully electric vehicles are expected to be widely available in the near future.

> Plan your vehicle trips to combine a number of errands instead of making several separate trips.

> Advocate for laws, policies, and actions that will reduce the risks associated with motor vehicles: lower speed limits, traffic calming, increased urban density, insurance premiums based on the distance driven, and infrastructure that favors walking, cycling, and public transit.

Radiation

We can be exposed to radiation from both natural and man-made sources. Most of the average person's exposure comes from natural sources—the sun (ultraviolet, or UV, radiation), geologic formations containing radioactive elements such as uranium (which produces radon as it decays), and cosmic radiation (from outer space). Man-made sources of radiation exposure include nuclear power plants, nuclear waste, x-rays, medical treatments, power lines, microwave ovens, and wireless transmissions such as WiFi and cell phones. Among the man-made sources, medical treatments such as radiation therapy for cancer make up the lion's share of exposure for most people, with nuclear accidents such as Chernobyl providing an important exception.

UV

The sun is a mind-boggling 150 million kilometers (90 million miles) from Earth (the precise distance varies because the Earth's orbit around the sun is elliptical). Sunlight travels at the speed of light, about 300,000 kilometers (more than 185,000 miles) per second, taking slightly more than eight minutes to reach us. By comparison, if you drove at 100 kilometers per hour (60 miles per hour) every hour of every day it would take you more than 170 years to drive that distance. Despite the incredible distance, exposure to sunlight can still cause adverse health effects in a brief span of time. Sunlight is a double-edged sword, offering important health benefits but also posing serious health risks unless precautions are taken.

Sunlight is a double-edged sword, offering important health benefits but also posing serious health risks

Exposure to sunlight is essential to good health because it allows your body to produce vitamin D, a nutrient needed to absorb calcium. Vitamin D helps maintain healthy bones and may even reduce the risk of some types of cancer. Unfortunately, because of damage to the Earth's protective ozone layer caused by a group of man-made chemicals, including CFCs, higher levels of harmful UV radiation are reaching the planet's surface and harming both human health and the environment.

There are two types of UV radiation—UVA and UVB. UVA radiation can cause premature aging of the skin and also harm the human immune system. Excessive exposure to UVB radiation can cause sunburn, skin cancer and other skin disorders, cataracts (which can lead to blindness) and other forms of eye damage, and reduced efficiency of the human immune system. Unprotected skin can be damaged in as little as fifteen minutes, yet it may take up to twelve hours for the full extent of a sunburn to become visible. While clouds filter UV radiation, they do not block it.

Melanoma is the most serious form of skin cancer because it can spread to other parts of the body. When detected at an early stage it is almost always treatable. Detecting melanoma early requires vigilance by you and your doctor. Non-melanoma skin cancers are more common but are rarely fatal.

Australia has the highest rate of skin cancer in the world; over 300,000 new cases of non-melanoma skin cancer and over 6,000 new melanoma cases are reported annually. This can be explained by the predominantly fair-skinned outdoors-loving population, the often cloud-free sky, and high levels of UV radiation. Skin cancer is the most common form of cancer in the U.S., with roughly 1 million new non-melanoma cases, 50,000 new melanoma cases, and 8,000 deaths annually. Close to a thousand Canadians die of melanoma annually, while approximately 4,000 new cases are diagnosed.

Detecting melanoma early requires vigilance by you and your doctor

Tens of thousands of North Americans are diagnosed with cataracts every year. In the U.S., cataract rates are projected to rise by 1.3% to 6.9% annually in the years ahead because of an aging population and ozone depletion (see page 154). This could amount to as many as 830,000 new cases in the U.S. by 2050, with costs to the health care system of almost $3 billion.

WHAT YOU CAN DO

> Avoid direct exposure to the sun during the middle of the day, especially in summer, and whenever the local UV index is high (see below). The UV index is used in weather forecasts around the world. Be particularly careful when you are in tropical regions and at higher elevations, where radiation is stronger.

HEALTHY AGING AND THE ENVIRONMENT ≪

AUSTRALIA, CANADA, AND the U.S. are each experiencing a dramatic demographic shift to an older population, with the number of senior citizens expected to almost double by 2030. Partly as a result of this, industrialized societies are grappling with a rapid increase in chronic age-related illnesses such as cancer, diabetes, and cardiovascular disease. Unless we move from a reactive, treatment-based model of medicine to a preventive model, the stress on health care systems will be intolerable. Vital elements of a preventive approach that permits healthy aging include a nutritious diet, regular physical and mental activity, and social support from family, friends, and community. As well, throughout life we all need to avoid exposure to environmental health hazards, including toxic chemicals and physical dangers such as radiation.

There is much to be learned from the people of Okinawa, Japan, who lead the world in life expectancy and the proportion of individuals living beyond a hundred years. Okinawans experience significantly lower rates of prostate and breast cancer, cardiovascular disease, and dementia. They are active daily, have a positive, relaxed attitude toward life, and eat low-calorie diets rich in vegetables, fiber, and healthy fats, including omega-3 fatty acids.

One of the most important quality-of-life determinants as you age is a healthy brain. Exposure to toxic chemicals can increase the risk of many diseases and conditions relevant to an aging population, including neurodegenerative disorders. Lead, certain pesticides, and air pollution are all linked to increased risk of Alzheimer's disease and Parkinson's disease. Logically, if we eliminate these poisonous substances from our air, food, water, and consumer products, we will see a decrease in these devastating diseases. For more information, see www.agehealthy.org.

UV Index

EXPOSURE CATEGORY	RANGE
LOW Minimal sun protection required for normal activity. Cover up, wear a hat, sunglasses, and sunscreen if outside for one hour or more.	2 OR LESS
MODERATE Sun protection required. Cover up, wear a hat, sunglasses, and sunscreen if outside for thirty minutes or more. Look for shade around midday.	3 TO 5
HIGH Full sun protection required. Cover up, wear a hat, sunglasses, and sunscreen. Reduce time in the sun between 11 a.m. and 4 p.m., and seek shade.	6 TO 7
VERY HIGH Extra precautions required. Unprotected skin burns and is damaged very quickly. Use sun protection, avoid time in the sun between 11 a.m. and 4 p.m., and seek shade.	8 TO 10
EXTREME Maximum precautions required. Unprotected skin burns and is damaged in minutes. Use sun protection, avoid time in the sun between 11 a.m. and 4 p.m., and seek shade.	11 OR HIGHER

www.msc-smc.ec.gc.ca/education/uvindex/who_newstd2_e.html

> When you are outside, use sun protection, including clothing, a hat with a wide brim, and good-quality sunglasses. Shade, whether from trees, buildings, or umbrellas, also offers good protection from the sun.

> Use sunscreen with a sufficiently high sun protection factor (SPF) to protect your skin (at least SPF 30 for fair-skinned individuals), and ensure that the brand you choose addresses both UVA and UVB radiation (see page 157). Apply up to thirty minutes before going outside and apply generously, as sunscreens only work effectively if applied in sufficient quantities. Re-apply as directed on the label. Studies show that most people use only half of the amount of sunscreen required, meaning they get only half of the protection available.

> Use extra caution when working, playing, or traveling on water, snow, ice, or sand, as reflective surfaces can increase your exposure to radiation and exacerbate sunburn.

> Be on the lookout for changes in the condition of your skin over time, particularly a mole that changes shape, size, or color, or the appearance of new bumps, nodules, or red scaly patches. Consult a doctor to determine if these are early warning signs for skin cancer.

> Avoid sunlamps and tanning salons.

> Do not look directly at the sun, particularly through binoculars, telescopes, and similar optical instruments. Looking at a partial solar eclipse (when the moon passes in front of the sun) is especially dangerous because the eye's pupil expands in the temporary darkness. The amount of light hitting retinal cells exposed to the partially blocked sun is ten times the amount that would occur while looking at the sun under normal conditions. This health hazard is particularly insidious because you feel no pain, yet your vision may be permanently impaired by blind spots.

> Push your government to expedite the phase-out of all remaining chemicals that deplete the Earth's vital ozone layer. While international agreements have produced tremendous progress in reducing releases

>> VITAMIN D AND THE
SUNSCREEN CONTROVERSY

THERE IS AN ongoing debate about whether it is better to wear sunscreen and protect yourself from UV radiation or to work on your tan and enjoy the benefits of vitamin D. As noted earlier, vitamin D is vital to healthy bones and it may also prevent osteoporosis and some immune system diseases. There is no doubt that the risk of skin cancer from exposure to UV radiation is real. Fortunately, there is a way out of this quandary: wear sunscreen and practice sun-smart behavior while obtaining your vitamin D through food and supplements.

You can get vitamin D from salmon, sardines, and other types of fish, cod liver oil, shiitake mushrooms, and egg yolks. Some foods—fortified milk, orange juice, yogurt, and cheese—have added vitamin D. As well, there are prescription and over-the-counter vitamin D supplements that come as pills, capsules, and liquids.

Currently, most governments recommend consuming at least 200 IU (international units) of vitamin D daily, and propose higher amounts for breastfed infants (400 IU per day) and people older than 50 (400 IU per day) or 70 (600 IU per day). Many scientists and doctors believe that government recommendations for vitamin D should be revised upward in light of recent information. Experts generally agree that 1,000 IU of vitamin D will provide additional health benefits without raising concerns about consuming too much.

of ozone-depleting substances, some industries are dragging their heels. A notorious example is methyl bromide, an ozone-depleting pesticide used to grow strawberries. This is a good reason to buy organic strawberries or strawberries from local farmers who refuse to use this nasty chemical.

Other Sources of Radiation

Extremely low frequency radiation is produced by power lines and, to a lesser extent, by wiring within buildings and some electrical appliances. Research indicates that there is an association between living close to power lines and the risk of childhood cancers, particularly leukemia. A recent British study found that children living within 600 meters of power lines faced an increased risk of 23% for leukemia, while children living within 200 meters (roughly 200 yards) of power lines faced an increased risk of 69%. As well, a portion of the population seems to suffer from electro-hypersensitivity—an allergic reaction to the electromagnetic fields produced by cell phones, appliances, power lines, and other electrical devices.

Research indicates that there is an association between living close to power lines and the risk of childhood cancers, particularly leukemia

Cell phones and cell phone antennas produce radiofrequency radiation. Some studies have linked heavy cell phone use to brain cancer (tumors on the side of the head where the phone is held), although results are not conclusive. Nevertheless, health authorities in the U.K., Germany, France, Finland, and Sweden now recommend that people exercise caution in using cell phones. In particular, European public health agencies recommend that parents limit their children's use of cell phones and are moving to prohibit cell phone advertising aimed at children. France recently announced plans to ban cell phones from primary schools.

X-ray radiation is commonly used in medicine to diagnose injuries and illness. Generally, the medical benefits of x-rays outweigh the risks, and advances in imaging technology allow patients to receive lower doses of radiation than were common in the past.

> If you are concerned about extremely low frequency radiation from power lines and you have children, avoid living within 600 meters (600 yards) of power lines.

> Do not drive or cycle while talking on a cell phone.

> When speaking on a cell phone, keep calls short. For lengthier conversations, use a hands-free headset or a landline.

> Do not insist on an x-ray if your doctor feels one isn't warranted. When an x-ray is warranted, ask your doctor if using an alternative imaging technology—such as ultrasound, magnetic resonance imaging, or thermography—is appropriate. Always make sure you are provided with a protective apron or other shield during an x-ray examination.

Environmental Noise

Noise, generally defined as unwanted sound, is an underappreciated environmental problem. Only recently have we begun to recognize that noise is a serious health hazard and not merely a nuisance. Like toxic chemicals, environmental noise is everywhere in today's industrialized societies: outdoors we are exposed to the roar of traffic while indoors we hear the constant hum of computers and other electronic items. Noise is also like toxic chemicals in that it is imposed on us by others, against our will and without our consent, in ways that we often have little control over or remedy against.

When you are exposed to noise, the ear's sensitivity level naturally decreases in order to protect your hearing, meaning that you will hear only sounds louder than a certain level. This change can be temporary (normally recovery occurs in less than twenty-four hours), chronic, or permanent. Millions of people in the U.S., Canada, and Australia suffer from noise-induced hearing loss. Sources of damaging noise include motor vehicles, lawn mowers, airplanes, helicopters, and construction equipment. Noise can adversely affect both our physical and mental health—something the Greeks recognized as early as 600 BCE, when they banned the hammering of metal within city limits. Similarly, the Romans banned the use of chariots at night because of the clattering of the wheels on paving stones.

Exposure to excessive noise can contribute to sleep disturbance, stress, headaches, high blood pressure, sexual impotence, mental illness, cardiovascular disease, changes in hormone levels, and a weakened immune system. Noise can also interfere with reading and problem solving, which affects performance at work and school, and cause irritability, which can change social behavior. Some individuals are particularly sensitive to certain kinds of noise and suffer severe impacts on their quality of life as a result.

Sources of damaging noise include motor vehicles, lawn mowers, airplanes, helicopters, and construction equipment

Sounds exceeding 85 decibels may cause slight, temporary hearing loss, while sounds louder than 100 decibels can cause permanent hearing loss. Noise is a common occupational hazard in many workplaces but can also be problematic in the home environment. Home shop tools, especially saws and drills, can generate noise of up to 110 decibels, explaining why the average twenty-five-year-old carpenter has the hearing of a fifty-year-old. Certain sources of noise, such as firearms, vacuum cleaners, and nail guns, produce impulse peaks that exacerbate the risk of hearing loss because the ear's protective mechanism does not have time to respond. Jet engines, motorcycles, subways, rock concerts, and personal media players can also produce unsafe levels of noise. It is important to appreciate that noise can have adverse effects even at levels too low to cause physical damage to hearing. Certain sounds can disturb sleep or raise blood pressure when they are inappropriate for a particular time or place (e.g., flights landing at an airport in the middle of the night or rock music in a cemetery).

WHAT YOU CAN DO

> Reduce your exposure to noise. For example, trade in your gas or electric lawn mower for a manual or push mower and enjoy the additional benefits of saving money, creating less pollution, and getting more exercise. Whenever possible, avoid close proximity to firearms, firecrackers, Jet Skis, leaf blowers, loud motorcycles, and other sources of excessive noise.

> Be a responsible consumer. Look for a noise rating when buying recreational equipment, children's toys, household appliances, and power tools. Choose quieter models, especially for equipment that you use often or operate close to your ears, such as a hair dryer. If there is no noise rating, contact the manufacturer and ask for one.

> Wear ear protection (earplugs or earmuffs) when using loud tools and appliances, traveling on loud vehicles, or listening to loud music. Hearing protection devices can be bought at most pharmacies and hardware stores.

> Keep the volume down when listening to your iPod or other personal media player.

> Communicate your concerns about noise to neighbors, businesses, and local governments. There is a widespread lack of education and understanding about the dangers of noise. Governments have a role to play in mandating quieter vehicles, tools, and appliances as well as regulating and enforcing ambient noise levels. See www.nonoise.org for a broad range of educational materials related to noise.

Advice for Parents

As is the case with chemical and biological hazards, children are the most vulnerable members of society when it comes to physical hazards. Protect your children's health by taking these steps:

> Always use appropriate safety equipment when driving with infants or children. Rely on child and booster seats that meet legal requirements and use them according to the manufacturer's instructions.

> Protect infants and children from UV radiation. This is vital because prolonged or repeated exposure to direct sunlight at a young age increases the risk of skin cancer later in life. Babies up to six months of age should not be exposed to direct sunlight at all. Sunscreen should not be used on babies, and an extra effort should be made to find a nontoxic brand for young children (see Chapter 6). Australia urges parents and teachers to ensure that all children wear hats to protect themselves from sunlight.

> Ensure children use cell phones primarily in emergency situations and not for daily calls.

> Protect the ears of children who are too young to protect themselves from excessive noise.

Wrap-up

Physical hazards have been widely recognized in the workplace for years but are only now gaining the wider recognition they deserve as serious threats to human health. As always, it is important to place risks in context. Rather than fearing exposure to radiation through a nuclear accident or nuclear war, you should consider the likelihood of exposure to radiation from more mundane sources, such as the sun (UV) and bedrock (radon). A few simple actions can significantly diminish the health risks posed by physical environmental hazards.

Avoid Physical Hazards

> Reduce your use of motor vehicles.

> Practice sun-smart behavior.

> Use cell phones sparingly, and with a headset for extended conversations.

> If you have young children or are planning to start a family, avoid living within 600 meters of power lines.

> Wear ear protection when exposed to loud noises.

8 ADVOCATE FOR A HEALTHY ENVIRONMENT

*To know that even one life has breathed easier
because you have lived, that is to have succeeded.*

Ralph Waldo Emerson

ALTHOUGH THIS BOOK outlines many practical steps you can take to protect your health, the burden of avoiding environmental hazards should not fall exclusively on the shoulders of individuals. Millions of people lack the time, knowledge, and resources required to protect themselves and their families from avoidable environmental risks. The most vulnerable people in our society are the most likely to be exposed to environmental hazards that are beyond their control. A triple-E approach to protecting environmental health—effective, efficient, and equitable—requires stronger government policies and major changes to business practices.

The U.S. Institute of Medicine, the Commission on the Future of Health Care in Canada, and the World Health Organization have all urged governments to pay greater attention and allocate more resources to environmental health. Stronger environmental policies and greener business practices could save thousands of lives every year in wealthy industrialized nations, prevent countless illnesses, help relieve the pressure on overloaded health care systems, make the economy more resilient, and improve the quality of our lives. Despite these potential benefits, governments and corporations in Australia, Canada, and the U.S. lag far behind their European counterparts in protecting human health from environmental hazards. Public pressure, applied creatively and relentlessly by citizens like you, is the only way to persuade politicians and business leaders to close this environmental health gap. While it may seem quixotic to imagine that a single person can change the world, the reality is that individuals do make a difference.

The most vulnerable people in our society are the most likely to be exposed to environmental hazards that are beyond their control

Consider the stories of some environmental health heroes. Rachel Carson was a pioneering environmental health advocate. Her 1962 book *Silent Spring*, which blew the whistle on the devastation wrought by pesticides, was a wake-up call not only in the U.S. but around the world. Carson wrote "If the Bill of Rights contains no guarantees that a citizen shall be secure against lethal poisons distributed either by private individuals or by public officials, it is surely only because our forefathers, despite their considerable wisdom and foresight, could conceive of no such problem." Lois Gibbs became an environmental health activist after investigating a series of illnesses that afflicted her seven-year-old son. She discovered that his elementary school and their entire neighborhood of Love Canal in Niagara Falls, New York, had been built on a hazardous waste dump. Gibbs' passionate advocacy led to the enactment of the Comprehensive Environmental Response, Compensation, and Liability Act, a law that requires the identification and restoration of toxic waste sites throughout the United States. Elizabeth May, a lawyer and leader of Canada's Green Party, has worked tirelessly on many issues, including an ongoing attempt to secure the full cleanup of Canada's most notorious toxic site, the Sydney Tar Ponds in Nova Scotia. Eileen Kampakuta Brown and Eileen Wani Wingfield are Aboriginal elders from Australia who worked to prevent a nuclear waste dump from being located in their traditional territory. During the 1950s and 1960s,

Brown and Wingfield witnessed the devastation caused by nuclear weapons testing in the Australian outback. Driven by their desire to protect the wild desert and groundwater their people depend on, these women led a successful campaign against further contamination and won the prestigious Goldman Prize for their efforts.

Erin Brockovich was a file clerk at a law firm when she stumbled across medical records suggesting that residents of Hinkley, California, suffered from unusually poor health. Brockovich eventually led a legal battle against the corporation that contaminated Hinkley's drinking water with hexavalent chromium, leading to a $333 million settlement, the cleanup of the contamination, and the award-winning movie starring Julia Roberts. Devra Davis grew up in Donora, Pennsylvania, where thousands of Americans became ill and dozens died because of terribly polluted air caused by local industries. Davis became a scientist and dedicated her career to pressing for stronger laws and policies to protect public health from environmental threats. Theo Colborn was a pharmacist before returning to school and earning a PhD in zoology at the age of fifty-eight. Colborn's ground-breaking research and her book, *Our Stolen Future*, propelled the issue of endocrine-disrupting chemicals onto the public stage, forcing governments to start studying and regulating these substances. It is now widely acknowledged that low-dose exposures to some industrial chemicals can disrupt human hormone systems and inflict environmental damage.

For each of these individuals who earned fame in the field of environmental health, there are millions more who have contributed to a healthier planet through grassroots efforts to clean up a beach or a community; stop corporate polluters from poisoning air, water, food, and land; or persuade governments to enact and enforce stronger environmental laws. As citizens, each of us has a vital role to play in convincing government and industry to be better stewards of human and ecological health and to behave in ways that protect our fundamental right to live in a clean environment.

Speak Up

Take one of the many opportunities available to voice your concerns about environmental impacts on human health. It might be easiest to start by talking about these issues with family, friends, neighbors, co-workers, teammates, fellow churchgoers, and others in your social circle. Listen to their concerns, and share your own. Discuss some of the solutions identified in this book. We tend to place greater trust in the people close to us than in the media, politicians, corporations, or other sources of information.

You could also raise environmental health issues with your doctor and other health professionals. It may come as a surprise that the majority of doctors and nurses lack specific training or expertise in the field of environmental threats to health. Despite this gap in their education, most health professionals understand that there are important connections between the well-being of people and the health of the planet. By talking about your environmental concerns you can help educate those in the field of health care. Consider giving a copy of this book to medical professionals that you meet, and urge them to lobby their professional associations to push for higher standards and a more preventive, precautionary approach to environmental health.

Communicate directly with elected representatives, civil servants, and businesses

You can also communicate directly with elected representatives, civil servants, and businesses. Whether you are pressing government for stronger laws and policies to protect people's health from environmental hazards or urging a corporation to clean up its act, you should start at the bottom *and* go straight to the top. Starting at the bottom means contacting a local politician or the manager of a local store to express your concerns. Going straight to the top means voicing your opinion to the president, the prime minister, governors, senators, members of Parliament, health ministers, environment ministers, mayors, and CEOs. Even though you probably won't receive a personal response, this doesn't mean you are not having an effect. In fact, governments and corporations survey public opinion regularly and keep close tabs on messages from voters and customers. Taking action to express your opinion has a much larger impact than you might imagine. Bureaucrats, politicians, and corporate executives know that for every letter or phone call they receive, dozens or hundreds more people share the same view but haven't taken the time to write or call. Form letters, postcards, and generic email messages have less impact than handwritten letters (see page 168), telephone calls, and face-to-face conversations.

You can share your views broadly by:

> Writing letters to the editors of newspapers and magazines.
> Calling radio programs.
> Posting messages or videos on the Internet.
> Writing your own blog.
> Creating your own website.
> Using social networking sites such as Twitter and Facebook.

Cast Your Ballot

Voting is both a right and a responsibility, and despite the pervasive changes associated with globalization, governments still exert tremendous influence over our lives. In particular, governments have the power to do many positive things to protect our health from environmental hazards, such as banning certain substances and products; ensuring clean air, clean water, and safe food; enforcing environmental laws against polluters; monitoring our body burdens; and providing information to citizens through mandatory product labeling and regular reports on environmental health. If your present political representatives are unable or unwilling to protect public health from environmental hazards, then vote the rascals out. Use your clout as a citizen to elect ecologically literate political leaders who understand that a precautionary

LETTER-WRITING TIPS, CONTACT INFORMATION, AND SAMPLE LETTER

> Be passionate but polite.

> Be brief (no more than two pages).

> Write to the right person.

> Make a clear and specific request.

> Ask for a response.

CONTACT INFORMATION

Prime Minister of Canada
80 Wellington Street
Ottawa, ON K1A 0A2

Email address:
pm@pm.gc.ca
Phone: 613-992-4211
Fax: 613-941-6900

To contact other elected
representatives in Canada,
see http://canada.gc.ca/
directories-repertoires/
direct-eng.html#mp.

President of the United States
c/o the White House
1600 Pennsylvania
Avenue NW
Washington, DC 20500

Email address:
President@whitehouse.gov or
Comments@whitehouse.gov
Phone: 202-456-1111 or
202-456-1414
Fax: 202-456-2461

To contact other elected
representatives in the U.S.,
see www.senate.gov,
www.house.gov, or
www.vote-smart.org.

Prime Minister of Australia
PO Box 6022
House of Representatives
Canberra, ACT 2600

Email: www.pm.gov.au/
contact/index.cfm
Phone: 02-6277-7700
Fax: 02-6273-4100

To contact other elected
representatives in Australia,
see www.aph.gov.au/library/
tutorial/contact.htm.

SAMPLE LETTER ON AIR POLLUTION

Dear President/Prime Minister:

I'm concerned about your government's failure to adequately protect people from air pollution. Reports from medical experts make it clear that dirty air continues to take a heavy toll on human health in this country, with thousands of deaths and millions of illnesses linked to pollutants in the air we breathe. Health problems caused by air pollution include cancer, heart disease, and respiratory illnesses. To make matters worse, these adverse effects disproportionately harm the most vulnerable members of our society— children and the elderly. For a nation with our level of wealth and technological prowess, surely this is an intolerable situation.

Respected health and environmental organizations have recommended three actions and I endorse them as well:

1. Strengthen and enforce standards for air quality, especially for particle pollution and ozone.

2. Change tax policies to discourage pollution and toxic releases, while reducing the tax burden on positive activities such as employment and investment.

3. Invest in planning and infrastructure that favors walking, cycling, public transit, and zero-emission vehicles.

These policies have a proven record of success in many nations. Please keep me informed about your government's efforts to clean the air, improve our health, and enhance our quality of life.

Sincerely,

Name
Address

approach is urgently required. Speak out at all-candidates meetings, or get involved with a political candidate or party. Ironically, voter turnout is lowest at the municipal level despite the fact that local politicians have the most direct effect on our everyday lives and environment. Vote every time you get the chance!

Harness the Power of Your Money

The ways that you spend and invest your money can have significant positive effects. Businesses will move quickly to green their products and operations when they perceive an impact on, a threat to, or the potential to improve their bottom line. You can use your power as a consumer to support businesses that are leaders in environmental responsibility and withdraw your support from the laggards. Stop buying products from companies that create harmful products or use hazardous chemicals, and inform them of your concerns with a quick email or letter.

Stop buying products from companies that create harmful products or use hazardous chemicals

Investing in companies that have a track record of corporate social responsibility makes more sense than allowing your savings to contribute to environmental destruction. As an added bonus, studies indicate that investing in socially and environmentally responsible corporations can provide a higher return on investment. Several websites offer excellent resources on socially responsible investing, including www.socialfunds.com. In Canada, see www.socialinvestment.ca. In the U.S., see www.socialinvest. org. In Australia, see www.responsibleinvestment.org. Similarly, you can transfer your bank accounts to a financial institution with a reputation for environmental leadership, and there are credit cards that donate money to green groups every time you make a purchase.

Multiply Your Impact

There is only so much an individual can do alone. Fortunately, there are some outstanding nongovernmental organizations engaged in the struggle for a cleaner, greener, healthier world. The more supporters these groups can enlist, the more influence they are able to wield with governments and industry. You can assist these organizations financially (by donating money or assets, or by making a bequest in your will) or by volunteering your time and energy to help them achieve their goals. Your financial support will be deeply appreciated and in most cases you will also receive a tax credit. The following organizations have excellent reputations.

Canada
- Canadian Association of Physicians for the Environment: www.cape.ca
- Canadian Cancer Society: www.cancer.ca
- Canadian Lung Association: www.lung.ca
- Canadian Partnership for Children's Health and the Environment: www.healthyenvironmentforkids.ca
- David Suzuki Foundation: www.davidsuzuki.org
- Ecojustice: www.ecojustice.ca
- Environmental Defence: www.environmentaldefence.ca
- Heart and Stroke Foundation of Canada: www.heartandstroke.ca
- Toxic Free Canada: www.toxicfreecanada.ca
- Waterkeeper Alliance: www.waterkeepers.ca

U.S.
- American Cancer Society: www.cancer.org
- American Heart Association: www.americanheart.org
- American Lung Association: www.lungusa.org

- Breast Cancer Fund: www.breastcancerfund.org
- Center for Health, Environment, and Justice: www.chej.org
- Earthjustice: www.earthjustice.org
- Environmental Working Group: www.ewg.org
- Healthy Child, Healthy World: www.healthychild.org
- Natural Resources Defense Council: www.nrdc.org
- Physicians for Social Responsibility: www.psr.org
- Waterkeeper Alliance: www.waterkeeper.org

Australia
- Australian Conservation Foundation: www.acfonline.org.au
- Australian Lung Foundation: www.lungfoundation.com.au
- Cancer Council Australia: www.cancer.org.au/home.htm
- Clean Up Australia: http://cleanup.org.au
- Doctors for the Environment Australia: http://dea.org.au/
- National Heart Foundation of Australia: www.heartfoundation.com.au
- National Toxics Network: http://ntn.org.au/

Learn More

This book presents just a fraction of the information available on environmental hazards. There is a staggering amount of information out there, and it can be difficult to separate fact from fiction (see page 175). Bear in mind that information is only as reliable as its source. Government websites often have good basic information, but are inclined to describe today's air, water, food, and consumer products as "safe" when experience proves that such broad assurances are false. As for information from industry, the warning "buyer beware" definitely applies. Many major industries and corporations have a long history of lies and deceit when it comes to the health and environmental consequences of their products and processes. Nongovernmental organizations can offer useful information but are sometimes selective, focusing primarily on evidence that supports their predetermined advocacy position.

The following Internet sources are highly recommended:

- Environmental Health News (www.EnvironmentalHealthNews.org) sifts through hundreds of newspapers and magazines daily to bring you the latest stories involving human health and the environment.

- Environmental Health Perspectives (www.ehponline.org) is a free online science journal exclusively dedicated to exploring the connections between health and the environment.

- PubMed (www.ncbi.nlm.nih.gov/pubmed) is a service offered by the U.S. National Library of Medicine and the National Institutes of Health that allows you to search online through hundreds of medical journals for articles on a specific topic.

- EcoHealth (www.ecohealth.net) is a journal published by the International Association for Ecology and Health.

The following outstanding books on human health and the environment are also recommended:

- E. Chivian and A. Bernstein, eds., *Sustaining Life: How Human Health Depends on Biodiversity* (Oxford University Press, 2008).

- D. Michaels, *Doubt Is Their Product: How Industry's Assault on Science Threatens Your Health* (Oxford University Press, 2008).

- D. Suzuki and A. McConnell, *The Sacred Balance: Rediscovering Our Place in Nature* (Greystone, 1997).

- T. Colborn, D. Dumanoski, and J.P. Myers, *Our Stolen Future: Are We Threatening Our Intelligence, Fertility, and Survival—A Scientific Detective Story* (Penguin, 1997).

See the Resources section at the end of this book for more recommendations.

Boycott the Bad Actors

There are some industries and companies that demonstrate a persistent disregard for human health and the environment. Industries that have wrought havoc for decades include the motor vehicle industry, the petroleum and coal industries, the asbestos industry, the chemical industry, and the lead industry. Examples of unrepentant anti-environmental companies include Exxon Mobil, notorious for financing bogus studies that deny the reality of climate change; Dole Food, whose use of the pesticide dibromochloropropane in Latin America (after it was banned in the U.S. for sterilizing men) caused lasting damage to the health of agricultural workers; and General Motors, the motor vehicle manufacturer that conspired to dismantle American public transit systems powered by electricity, fought against tougher fuel efficiency and air pollution standards, sabotaged its own electric car project in the 1990s, and began selling gas-guzzling Hummers and other large SUVs instead. Boycotts are a powerful way to increase awareness of this kind of corporate irresponsibility. They can serve more than one purpose, both raising the profile of important issues and persuading businesses to improve their environmental record. Green America offers an excellent boycott organizer's guide, available free from www.boycotts.org.

> Boycotts are a powerful way to increase awareness of corporate irresponsibility

Fight for Your Rights

One of the most important demands you can make is that governments recognize your right to live in a healthy environment. If this basic human right is not in your national constitution, it should be, since constitutions reflect the core values of a society and establish the most important rules governing the legal system. Unfortunately, the constitutions of Canada, the U.S., and Australia are silent on the matter of protecting the environment. In contrast, the constitutions of more than 80 nations recognize

EVERYONE KNOWS THAT the tobacco industry lied, manipulated science, and deliberately deceived both the public and policymakers about the catastrophic health effects of smoking. Far fewer people are aware that the same strategy of deceit and denial—employing the same tactics, the same public relations firms, and even some of the same scientists—has been and is still used by many corporations and industries today. The list of toxic substances disingenuously defended by corporations is lengthy: asbestos, lead, CFCS, vinyl chloride, mercury, phthalates, beryllium, bisphenol A, benzene, chromium 6, polybrominated diphenyl ethers, pesticides, diacetyl, and benzidine dyes (used in textiles and leathers). The motor vehicle and fossil fuel industries used the identical approach to muddy the waters about air pollution and climate change.

The basic strategy involves distorting and misrepresenting science to create a false sense of uncertainty about whether a substance or product causes harm to human health or the environment. As a tobacco industry executive wrote in an infamous memo uncovered through litigation, "doubt is our product." The tactics used by industry and their accomplices include sponsoring studies that have predetermined favorable results; financing pseudo-scientific journals with authoritative-sounding titles that will publish studies of dubious merit; creating organizations whose names suggest they are legitimate community, health, or environmental groups when they are mere industry fronts; confounding regulators with reams of lengthy but bogus studies; and using litigation as a last ditch way to block regulation. By sowing seeds of doubt, industry is able to delay and often defeat proposed regulations intended to protect public health. For more information about these tactics, see www.DefendingScience.org.

the right to live in a healthy environment, and 140 constitutions impose a duty on governments to safeguard the environment. Constitutional recognition of the right to live in a healthy environment obligates governments, at all levels, to respect, protect, and fulfill that right. The right to a healthy environment includes three important procedural rights—access to information, participation in decision making, and access to justice. It is no coincidence that the nations with the best environmental records in the world—Sweden, Norway, Finland, and Switzerland—have strong constitutional provisions requiring protection of the environment. Nations that lag behind in environmental performance ratings—Canada, the U.S., and Australia—lack constitutional protection for the environment.

Unfortunately, the constitutions of Canada, the U.S., and Australia are silent on the matter of protecting the environment

Closely related to the right to live in a healthy environment is the right to know what chemicals and other hazards you may be exposed to on a daily basis. For years, laws have required employers to provide workers with comprehensive information about the toxic substances that they may be exposed to in the workplace. This is called a worker's "right to know" and has been partially extended to the general public through legislation requiring large companies to disclose their toxic releases into the air, water, and soil. Unfortunately, no similar rules apply to toxic substances in food or consumer products. Product labels on the majority of consumer items fail to disclose all ingredients, or else do so in microscopic print using language that requires a doctorate in chemistry to decipher. California and Europe are exceptions to this rule, as they require disclosure of ingredients that cause cancer or reproductive harm. Whether we are talking about cancer-causing chemicals in household cleaners, food made from genetically modified organisms, or products incorporating nanotechnology, the basic point is that citizens have a right to know what is in their air, water, food, and the products they buy.

Set the Bar High

Another key initiative involves insisting that environmental standards in your country be raised to meet or beat the highest standards in the world. Why should you, your family, friends, and neighbors be treated like second-class citizens? In terms of air quality, drinking water quality, rules governing contaminants in food, and the regulation of toxic substances in consumer products, Europe consistently sets higher standards than Canada, the U.S., or Australia. Here are a few examples:

- Unlike Canada, the U.S., and Australia, Europe prohibits the use of arsenic, antibiotics, and hormones in livestock to foster accelerated growth.
- European rules governing asbestos, phthalates, and brominated flame retardants are stronger than North American or Australian rules.
- Europe prohibits the use of many pesticides that continue to be permitted in Canada, the U.S., and Australia.
- Europe prohibits the use of many ingredients used in cosmetics and personal care products that continue to be allowed in Canada, the U.S., and Australia.

It's time for the rest of the industrialized world to catch up with the Europeans, who understand that protecting the environment means protecting ourselves.

Require Substitutes for Health-harming Chemicals

Every week there is more evidence connecting industrial chemicals and the by-products of burning fossil fuels to the epidemic of chronic diseases afflicting modern society, including cancer, neurological disorders, cardiovascular disease, respiratory illness, and reproductive problems. In response, Sweden pioneered a concept called substitution, requiring that safer substances replace hazardous ones wherever possible. The substitution principle is now the law throughout Europe.

Strong regulatory action can produce swift results. Children's blood lead levels dropped dramatically in nations where leaded gasoline was banned. From Dublin to Hong Kong, stronger air quality laws have produced declines in heart and lung disease. In another promising example, Swedish cancer experts believe that early regulatory action on pesticides and other toxic substances by the government of Sweden may have contributed to declining rates of some cancers. Sweden now plans to prohibit all products and processes containing or releasing carcinogens, mutagens, endocrine disruptors, reproductive toxicants, and the heavy metals lead, mercury, and cadmium by 2015. As well, Sweden is aiming to eliminate the use of fossil fuels in transportation by 2030, which will result in substantial health benefits as well as the obvious environmental dividends.

Shift the Burden of Proof

Currently, we consider chemicals innocent until proven guilty. Tens of thousands of industrial chemicals have entered the marketplace in recent decades without adequate testing for human or environmental health. Governments, independent scientists, and the public bear a heavy burden of proof in establishing beyond a reasonable doubt that these chemicals cause harm. In the rare cases where governments do apply the precautionary principle, corporations fight back aggressively. For example, Dow AgroSciences is suing Canada for millions of dollars under the North American Free Trade Agreement because the province of Quebec passed a law prohibiting the cosmetic and nonessential uses of pesticides, including the herbicide 2,4-D. Dow claims there is no conclusive scientific proof that 2,4-D harms human health, although numerous European nations have already banned it because of health and environmental concerns.

We'd be better off reversing our approach and considering chemicals harmful until there is enough evidence to suggest otherwise. People, not toxic chemicals, have rights. We should err on the side of caution, and place the onus on industry to prove beyond a reasonable doubt that a product and the chemicals it contains or releases are safe.

Extend Your Compassion

Even though there is still a long way to go in Canada, the U.S., and Australia, these nations have made progress in providing people with cleaner air and water, and reducing at least some environmental health risks. Developing nations, by contrast, face far more severe health problems associated with dirty air and water, and a host of toxic substances. There are still nations where leaded gasoline and lead paint continue to be used, where pesticides and other chemicals long since banned in wealthy nations are still permitted, and where environmental laws either do not exist or are rarely, if ever, enforced.

There are still nations where leaded gasoline and lead paint continue to be used

To protect public health worldwide, especially children's health, the world's wealthy nations urgently need to contribute more to aid efforts. Making the investments necessary to fulfill the UN's Millennium Development Goals (MDGs) by 2015 is an obvious starting point. These global goals include eradicating extreme poverty and hunger; achieving universal primary education; promoting gender equality and empowering women; reducing child mortality; improving maternal health; combating HIV/AIDS, malaria, and other preventable diseases; and halving the proportion of the population that lacks access to safe drinking water and basic sanitation. Achieving the MDGs will require the investment of US$150 to $200 billion per year through 2015, which sounds like a vast sum of money but is actually a drop in the bucket of a global economy approaching US$60 trillion. To their ongoing shame, the U.S., Canada, and Australia trail far behind leading European nations in levels of aid to developing nations. Other essential steps to protect global environmental health include reducing trade barriers that harm the economies of developing nations, and promoting the health, education, and economic opportunities of girls and young women.

In addition, the world urgently needs an agreement to rapidly phase out all nonessential uses of lead, mercury, and other substances that damage the brain of the fetus, infant, and young child during crucial stages of development. Solving the complex challenges of the coming decades will require the full intellectual capacity of future generations, undiminished by irreversible brain damage. There is some reason for optimism, especially with the U.S. government's recent decision to reverse its position opposing a global treaty on mercury that is under negotiation. However, approaching environmental health concerns one substance at a time is misguided because it would take centuries to negotiate international agreements to address thousands of hazardous substances.

Rapid action to save the ozone layer prevented a global health catastrophe and serves as a promising sign that we can solve other global environmental problems

A better approach would be to tackle groups of chemicals simultaneously. This strategy has worked in the past with both ozone-depleting chemicals and persistent organic pollutants. The Stockholm Convention on Persistent Organic Pollutants targets the so-called dirty dozen, twelve toxic substances that do not easily break down, are capable of building up in the environment (and in people), and pose severe threats to human health. Almost 150 nations are parties to the Stockholm Convention, meaning they are committed to eliminating the dirty dozen, and negotiations are ongoing about extending the agreement to cover additional substances. Similarly, nations of the world agreed upon the Montreal Protocol on Substances that Deplete the Ozone Layer in 1987, leading to dramatic reductions in the production, use, and release of CFCs and other chemicals that were destroying the Earth's protective ozone layer. Rapid action to save the ozone layer prevented a global health catastrophe and serves as a promising sign that we can solve other global environmental problems. Full implementation of the international agreements to protect the Earth's ozone layer is expected to provide the world with over $200 billion in net health and environmental benefits.

Wrap-up

One of our key duties as citizens is to help political and business leaders find the path to a prosperous, just, and sustainable future. We can provide enthusiastic encouragement where warranted and constructive criticism when necessary. We can demonstrate our support for strong leadership on health and environmental issues when marking our ballots, making our purchases, conversing with friends, and sitting at our computers. Just as each of the trillions of cells in our bodies seems tiny and insignificant on its own but is a part of a larger, wonderful, and mysterious whole, so too can each of us as individuals be a part of the large, wonderful, and organic movement for a sustainable future.

One person's vote can change the outcome of an election. One person's purchase can save a small business. One person's donation can push an environmental health campaign over the top. One person's letter can inspire a thousand more letters. Your understanding of environmental risks can be used to improve not only your health, but also the health of family, friends, and neighbors. Your timely intervention could make someone's day or save a child's life. Through your words and your actions, you can be a source of both information and inspiration.

Act for a Healthy Planet

> Speak up on behalf of cleaner, greener policies, practices, governments, and businesses.

> Vote and campaign for pro-environment politicians.

> Support businesses that respect environmental health, and boycott bad actors.

> Donate money, time, or both to nonprofit health and environment groups.

> Learn more about environmental health.

> Fight for your right to live in a healthy environment.

> Advocate for high standards to protect both health and the environment.

> Encourage businesses to substitute safer chemicals for hazardous ones.

> Shift the burden of proof to industry to demonstrate their products are safe.

> Call for policies and actions that help the citizens of developing nations.

9 HEALTHY PLANET, HEALTHY PEOPLE

Once people recognize how much is at stake with their health and lives,
and with the health and lives of their children, they will do everything
in their power to protect the global environment.

Eric Chivian, MD and Aaron Bernstein, MD,
editors of *Sustaining Life: How Human Health Depends on Biodiversity*

ASTRONOMERS HAVE IDENTIFIED roughly 350 exoplanets—
planets that are outside our solar system and orbiting stars other
than our sun. Estimates suggest there may be as many as 100 billion planets in our galaxy, and 100 billion galaxies in the universe. Despite intense
effort, technological advances, and much speculation about extrater-
restrials, no other planet that supports life has been identified. Earth,
with its habitable biosphere, may well be unique, indicating that we are
extraordinarily blessed to be able to call this planet home. Despite our
miraculous good fortune, humans take the Earth for granted, assuming
that the planet is so big, so bountiful, and so resilient that our material
demands, pollution, and waste could never cause serious damage on
a global scale. This assumption is no longer valid in a world of nearly
7 billion people in relentless pursuit of economic growth. We need to rad-
ically alter our relationship with the Earth in ways that restore its health
and ensure its continued well-being. This is the only way to guarantee
that our children and grandchildren will lead healthy and happy lives.

So far we've focused on the steps you can take to protect your health from direct threats posed by environmental hazards in air, food, water, and consumer products. However, there are two environmental crises that have potentially immense consequences for human health—climate change and declining biological diversity. Both crises are driven by the increasing human population and the ideology of limitless growth, which in turn leads to overconsumption. The global population is expected to surpass 7 billion in 2012, and UN projections estimate that there will be 9 billion or even 10 billion people living in 2050. For decades now, per capita consumption of energy and resources has climbed relentlessly upward, even in societies that are already wealthy. Successful, sustainable solutions will need to address population growth and overconsumption if we are to prevent a climate catastrophe and protect the diversity of life. The challenges are, admittedly, daunting, and will require an unprecedented international effort that combines ecological education, innovative public policies, technological breakthroughs, and substantial behavioral changes. On an individual level, taking action to reduce your contribution to climate change and to help protect biodiversity will also protect your health, your children's health, and the health of future generations.

> There are two environmental crises that have potentially immense consequences for human health—climate change and declining biological diversity

Although this book is about environmental threats to human health, it is essential to appreciate that the environment also plays a vital role in promoting human health. Ecosystems provide indispensable services that ensure a steady supply of fresh air, clean water, and wholesome food, as well as natural capital in the form of everything from forests to fisheries. In addition, contact with the natural world improves physical health, psychological well-being, and, perhaps most importantly, happiness.

Climate Change and Health

While it is clear that climate change is taking place and that human activities (mainly burning fossil fuels, clearing forests, and raising livestock) are to blame, there is uncertainty about the effects that climate change will have on human health in either the short or long run. Nevertheless, in 2009 the respected British medical journal *The Lancet* described climate change as "the biggest global health threat of the twenty-first century." Climate change is expected to contribute to more extreme weather events, heat deaths, chronic water shortages, changes in food production, increased levels of allergens, and the spread of infectious diseases. The World Health Organization estimates that climate change already causes 150,000 deaths and 5 million illnesses per year and projects a doubling of these figures by 2030. The heat wave that struck Europe in 2003 killed as many as thirty-five thousand people. More than a billion people are expected to face chronic water shortages in a few decades as precipitation patterns change and water supplies stored in glaciers and snowpacks decline. Australia is experiencing its worst drought in a thousand years, and precipitation levels in hard-hit southern Australia are projected to decline in coming decades. In 2009, the Murray River, which supplies drinking water to Adelaide and other cities, had the lowest flows in the 117 years on record. Infectious diseases, from malaria to West Nile virus, are spreading into new regions. West Nile virus arrived in New York City in 1999 and is now endemic across most of North America. The Asian tiger mosquito caused an outbreak of a tropical disease called Chikungunya in Italy in 2007. This marked the first Chikungunya outbreak outside tropical regions.

Climate change will also have impacts on food production. Increased frequency and severity of droughts are anticipated for the regions of Africa that already suffer from significant levels of malnutrition. The increased emphasis on biofuels as a cleaner substitute for fossil fuels has caused a shift in farming away from food crops to fuel crops, contributing to a spike in global food prices that hit poor people hardest. It is estimated that for every 1% increase in the price of staples such as rice, an additional 16 million people face elevated risks of hunger.

Perversely, the countries that have done the least to cause climate change (because they have produced far fewer tonnes of greenhouse gas emissions) are expected to suffer the largest impacts. Adverse health outcomes in developing countries that will worsen due to climate change include diarrhea, malaria, and fatalities caused by flooding, hurricanes, cyclones, and other extreme weather events. Tens of millions of environmental refugees could be created by climate change. For example, in Bangladesh, one of the world's poorest nations, millions of people live in coastal areas that are less than a meter above sea level. Small island nations, including the Maldives, Tuvalu, and Vanuatu, are actively looking for land in other countries because they anticipate being forced to resettle their entire populations.

Tens of millions of environmental refugees could be created by climate change

Biodiversity and Health

In much the same way that our well-being relies on a stable climate, we are dependent on the global web of natural diversity. According to Dr. E.O. Wilson of Harvard University, "Biodiversity matters profoundly to human health, and in almost every conceivable way." We depend on Nature for food, water, wood, and other renewable resources. The majority of pharmaceutical products and medicines are derived from or inspired by natural species, particularly plants. Taxol, a drug used to treat cancer patients, comes from the Pacific yew tree. Survival rates for childhood leukemia and Hodgkin's lymphoma have increased dramatically thanks to vincristine and vinblastine, two drugs derived from a plant called rosy periwinkle. Artemisinin is a drug used to fight malaria that comes from sweet wormwood, an endangered plant from central China. Several important antibiotics are derived from fungi found in tropical soils.

Animals also play a role in protecting human health. Important medicines derived from animals include an anticoagulant isolated from the saliva of the canine hookworm, and a hypertension drug inspired by the venom of the pit viper. Toxins produced by cone snails to defend themselves and paralyze their prey are being used to make pain medications and may be useful in treating degenerative neurological diseases such as Alzheimer's and Parkinson's. Polar bears may hold the secret to preventing loss of bone mass, treating kidney disease, and understanding the connection between obesity and type 2 diabetes. Despite scarcely moving during hibernation, polar bears do not experience bone loss. Despite not urinating for months, bears do not endure toxicity related to the buildup of urinary wastes, as humans do. Prior to hibernating for five or more months, polar bears become obese, yet they do not develop diabetes. If polar bears go extinct, they could take invaluable medical secrets with them.

That is precisely what happened with gastric brooding frogs, a remarkable species that was found only in undisturbed Australian rainforests. Female gastric brooding frogs were the only species that raised their young inside their stomachs. The female frogs swallowed their fertilized eggs, which hatched, grew into fully developed tadpoles, and were then vomited out into the world. Scientists believe that the tadpoles secreted a substance that prevented them from being digested by their mothers. This substance could have provided insights into treating peptic ulcers, a disease afflicting tens of millions of people. Sadly, gastric brooding frogs are now believed to be extinct.

Humans rely extensively on other species for biomedical research. Many of the basic building blocks of seemingly diverse and disparate species—molecules, cells, tissues, organs—are so similar that we can use them to better understand human physiology. We share hundreds of our estimated twenty-five thousand genes with bacteria, thousands with yeasts, almost half our genes with fruit flies, and even more with the common mouse. Examples of medical developments based upon animal research include anesthetics, antibiotics, vaccines, blood transfusions, and kidney dialysis.

The most comprehensive global assessment of the number of species on Earth estimates a total of 13 to 14 million species, yet fewer than 2 million species have been identified to date. Only a tiny fraction of those 2 million plants, animals, and microbes have been studied for their potential medical value. As Dr. Gro Harlem Brundtland, the former prime minister of Norway and director-general of the World Health Organization, stated, "The library of life is burning and we do not even know the titles of the books." Some of the species that are known to be important to human medicine are designated as threatened or endangered, including primates, bears, sharks, amphibians, horseshoe crabs, and cone snails.

Even less widely appreciated are the ecosystem services that Nature provides—services of incalculable value in protecting human health. Examples include the pollination of food crops by insects, the release of oxygen by trees and other plants, the storage and purification of water by wetlands, and the decomposition of waste by fungi and bacteria. Also vital are the global cycles of nutrients—nitrogen, phosphorous, and other elements—that are essential to life. Many of these invisible processes are taken for granted, yet ecosystems need to be healthy in order to provide these services. The UN's comprehensive Millennium Ecosystem Assessment concluded that 60% of the ecosystem services they evaluated—from fresh water and soil cycles to atmospheric stability and fisheries—are being degraded or used unsustainably. For example, bee populations are suffering rapid declines because of exposure to pesticides and infection by parasites. Bees pollinate food crops worth tens of billions of dollars, as well as myriad native plants relied upon by other species. Ecosystem services are so incredibly complex and take place on such a vast scale that it would be virtually impossible to replace them should ecosystems be irreparably damaged.

Damaged ecosystems and declines in biodiversity also contribute to changing patterns of infectious disease in humans (see page 190). While we tend to think of illnesses being passed on from person to person, the majority involve pathogens that live and multiply in other organisms before infecting people. We are exposed to these pathogens through insect bites (e.g., malaria and Lyme disease), contaminated food or water (e.g., salmonellosis and cryptosporidiosis), contact with the urine or feces of infected animals (e.g., hantavirus pulmonary syndrome), or bacteria that we inhale (e.g., tularemia, or rabbit fever). Activities such as deforestation, agriculture, urbanization, and water management can disturb ecosystems in ways that increase the risk of infectious disease. For example, West Nile virus is more likely to harm human health where the diversity of mosquito-eating insects and animals has declined, and where the diversity and populations of native bird species have declined. This is because native birds are poor hosts for some strains of the virus and the introduced birds that often replace native ones are good hosts, ensuring the spread of the disease. The implications are clear. Healthy ecosystems equal healthy people. And healthy ecosystems depend on people living more lightly on the earth.

Examples of medical developments based upon animal research include anesthetics, antibiotics, vaccines, blood transfusions, and kidney dialysis

Reducing Your Ecological Footprint

The challenges of climate change and declining biodiversity are large but not insurmountable. Solutions are either already available or are tantalizingly close, including clean, renewable sources of energy, buildings that produce as much energy as they use, zero-emission vehicles powered by electricity or hydrogen, compact cities that apply the principles of Smart Growth, low-impact high-quality lifestyles, and cradle-to-cradle products that produce nutrients for biological and technological systems instead of waste (see page 195). At an individual level, the most important thing you can do to reduce the adverse environmental effects of your lifestyle is to reduce your ecological footprint. Key choices that determine

ZOONOSES AND THE ENVIRONMENT «

ZOONOSES ARE DISEASES or infections that are transmitted from vertebrate animals to humans. Recent outbreaks of SARS (severe acute respiratory syndrome) and so-called bird or swine flu (infections caused by subtypes of influenza A viruses such as H5N1 and H1N1) illustrate the potential of microorganisms from animal reservoirs to adapt to human hosts. A wide variety of animal species—domesticated, feral, and wild—can act as reservoirs for these pathogens, which may be viruses, bacteria, parasites, or prions.

During recent decades, many previously unknown human infectious diseases have emerged from animal reservoirs, including HIV (human immunodeficiency virus) and Ebola and Nipah viruses. More than 75% of new, emerging, and re-emerging human diseases at the beginning of the twenty-first century are caused by pathogens originating from animals or products of animal origin.

Human influences, including global travel, are major factors in the emergence and spread of zoonotic diseases. The burgeoning human population and increasing levels of wealth lead to rising demand for meat and explosive growth in intensive livestock operations. The consequences can include large numbers of people and animals living in close proximity, damaged and disturbed natural habitats, and climate change. An example of this pattern is the outbreak of Nipah virus in Malaysia in 1999, when intensive pig farming intruded into the natural habitat of fruit bats carrying the virus. The pig population became infected, acted as the host, and eventually transmitted the virus to farmers, resulting in 105 deaths.

The outbreaks of SARS, bird flu, swine flu, and Nipah virus are a wake-up call for the world. They demonstrate the potential seriousness of emerging zoonotic diseases and how even countries with advanced public health systems may struggle to cope with such diseases.

the size of your ecological footprint include where you live, what you eat, how you travel, and what products you buy.

Home
> Choose a modestly sized home near family, friends, work, school, recreation, and public transit.
> Get a home energy audit and follow the energy-saving recommendations.
> Generate or purchase green electricity (e.g., solar, wind, biomass, or micro-hydro).

Food
> Choose healthy whole foods, produced locally and organically.
> Eat more plant-based foods and less meat, eggs, and dairy.
> Focus on improving the quality of the food you eat, and decreasing the quantity.

Travel
> Rely on green alternatives (walking, cycling, public transit, car-sharing, carpooling, telecommuting, and videoconferencing) whenever possible, rather than driving or flying.
> Stay close to home more often, especially for holidays (e.g., take "100-mile" vacations)
> Drive the smallest, most fuel-efficient vehicle that meets your needs, ideally an electric car or gas-electric hybrid.

Consumer Products
> Focus on the big picture—worry less about plastic bags and more about energy use and your overall ecological footprint.
> Buy less stuff, especially products containing toxic ingredients or components.

> Do not buy products that will end up in the garbage because they are not durable and can't be reused, recycled, or composted.

Citizenship
> Become an active citizen—vote, speak out about environmental issues, and support pro-environment politicians and businesses.

> Donate time and money to environmental organizations.

> Invest your money in socially responsible banks, companies, and other organizations.

Nature
> Spend more time outdoors, especially with children.

> Take back some of your time from work, TV, the Internet, and shopping (in effect, you'll be trading money for health and happiness).

Recap: How to Protect Your Health

When all is said and done, it is important to put environmental health challenges in perspective. First, there are personal factors that may pose a greater threat to your health—such as smoking, a poor diet, lack of exercise, and the use of drugs. Second, there are social factors that put some people at greater risk of ill health—poverty, lack of education, and unequal access to health services. Third, while the Bobby McFerrin approach to environmental health (don't worry, be happy) is obviously unwarranted, we need to recognize that our environmental health problems are relatively minor compared with the challenges facing developing nations. In poor countries, environmental hazards kill millions of children annually, and diseases that could be prevented or treated for mere pennies per child kill millions more.

While there is a large amount of information in this book, protecting your health from environmental hazards boils down to three critical steps:

1. Be aware of the environmental hazards you are likely to encounter and ignore those that pose little or no risk. Just as there is no point worrying about a grizzly bear attack if you are camping in Australia, there is no point worrying about a toxic substance that you are unlikely to be exposed to in your life.

2. Eliminate sources of hazards. When it comes to indoor air, food, and consumer products, there are simple steps you can take to completely eliminate certain environmental hazards from your life. For example, you can rid your home of lead, toxic cleaning products, and items that release volatile organic compounds. Similarly, if you refuse to use pesticides in your home or garden and eat primarily organic foods, then you effectively eliminate the main sources of exposure to this group of hazardous substances.

3. Limit your exposure. In some cases, it is impossible for individuals to eliminate the source of environmental hazards. For health threats posed by outdoor air, UV radiation, and drinking water, the solutions are not staying indoors twenty-four hours a day and drinking bottled water. Instead, you should use the knowledge gained from reading this book to make wise choices: determine when it is safe to spend time outdoors; practice sun-smart behavior; and decide whether you need to install a water treatment system in your home.

A Happy Ending

Having spent most of this book describing the health threats posed by environmental hazards—the toxic bullets we dodge every day—it is refreshing to close by focusing on the health benefits that the environment can provide. We are all healthier because of the biodiversity and ecosystem services described in this chapter, and because of the physical and psychological benefits we enjoy from spending time outside in natural settings. The value of happiness induced by contact with the natural world should never be underestimated.

Research demonstrates that contact with the natural world counteracts stress, decreases anxiety, and accelerates recovery from illness. One remarkable study found that hospital patients in beds facing windows that looked out on trees recuperated significantly faster and required less pain medication than patients in beds facing windows that looked out on a brick wall. Playing outside is especially vital for children, who need to spend time in natural settings to develop cognitive and motor skills. Access to green space and pleasant outdoor environments allows seniors to remain physically active, which ultimately extends their lives.

The value of happiness induced by contact with the natural world should never be underestimated

Contact with Nature provides so many mental and physical benefits that some experts are calling for it to be recognized and promoted as part of a public health strategy. One of the most important things you can do to improve your health and well-being is spend more time being active outdoors: running, walking your dog, playing sports, riding your bike, paddling or sailing a boat, digging in your garden, or swimming in a lake, ocean, or river. The possibilities are endless.

Yoga, meditation, tai chi, and other mind-body practices used to be regarded as suitable only for hippies and new-age gurus. Today there is compelling scientific evidence that these practices can improve your health and prevent disease. While it remains true that you cannot change your genes, you may be able to change the way your genes behave. For example, research has demonstrated that intensive lifestyle changes, including exercise and stress management techniques advocated by practitioners of integrative medicine, can "turn on" disease-preventing genes and "turn off" genes that promote diseases such as prostate cancer. These activities can be done outdoors and have virtually no environmental impact.

The deeper your connection to Nature and the more time you spend outdoors, the happier you are likely to be. Studies show that people who adopt environmentally friendly behaviors such as riding bicycles and

SCANDINAVIAN NATIONS ARE consistently at the top of global rankings for environmental protection, health care, and economic performance. In a recent comparison of seventeen wealthy nations, Sweden, Finland, and Norway ranked first, second, and third on environmental performance while Canada, Australia, and the U.S. finished at the very bottom of the rankings. The three Scandinavian nations also ranked higher on indicators of economic performance. Since 1990, Sweden's economy has grown by 48%, while greenhouse gas emissions have fallen by 9%, meaning Sweden went well beyond its Kyoto commitment. Scandinavian nations have remarkably generous social policies. In Sweden, university tuition is free, and each parent is entitled to 240 days of paid parental leave when a child is born. Norway and Sweden provide three to four times more financial assistance to the world's poorest countries than Australia, Canada, or the U.S.

The Scandinavians demonstrate that strong environmental policies create a virtuous circle of health, environmental, and economic benefits, leading to even more progressive policies. Their inspiring success demolishes the arguments used to block environmental progress: that ecological degradation is an inevitable by-product of human activity; that strong environmental policies will damage the economy; and that switching to greener lifestyles means sacrificing today's standard of living and returning to the misery of centuries past. In fact, there is no trade-off between a healthy environment and a prosperous economy. Such thinking is as outdated as believing in a flat Earth. Instead, Sweden, Norway, and Finland illustrate the compelling connections between a clean environment, lower health care costs, economic prosperity, and high quality of life.

recycling tend to be happier. These findings contradict the stereotype of the gloomy environmentalist, and provide evidence that following the advice in this book will not only improve your health, but will increase your level of happiness. Happy people live longer, healthier lives. People who report frequent happy feelings are less likely to suffer from stroke and cardiovascular disease, and live up to seven years longer than those who are less happy. Happy people are more productive at work and enjoy higher job satisfaction. Happiness is also inversely correlated with air pollution, so when the quantity of air pollutants goes down, the amount of happiness measured goes up. The bottom line is that health, happiness, and environmentally friendly behavior are complementary and mutually reinforcing.

The bottom line is that health, happiness, and environmentally friendly behavior are complementary and mutually reinforcing

Human beings are an incredible species, living on an extraordinary planet. Our fate is inextricably intertwined with the destiny of the natural world. The revelation that today's children may lead shorter, less healthy lives indicates that we are failing in one of our most sacred obligations—to leave the world we inherited from our parents in shape that is just as good, if not better, for our children. Our best and brightest scientists tell us that a healthy environment is a fundamental prerequisite for healthy people. We need to listen to their wisdom and act accordingly. We need to treat both the Earth and ourselves with newfound wonder, reverence, and respect. There is much more that each and every one of us could do to make our lives cleaner, greener, healthier, and happier. Our health, our children's health, and the future of life on Earth depend on it.

RESOURCES

1 Environmental Health 101

Government Sources of Information on Environmental Health

AUSTRALIA

- Department of the Environment, Water, Heritage and the Arts
  www.environment.gov.au

- Department of Health and Aging (Environmental Health)
  www.health.gov.au/internet/main/publishing.nsf/Content/
  portal-Environmental%20health

- Environmental Health Council http://enhealth.nphp.gov.au/

CANADA

- Chemical Substances Management
  www.chemicalsubstanceschimiques.gc.ca/en/

- Environment Canada www.ec.gc.ca

- Health Canada www.hc-sc.gc.ca/ewh-semt/index-eng.php

- Healthy Canadians www.healthycanadians.ca/index_e.html

- National Collaborating Centre for Environmental Health www.ncceh.ca

UNITED STATES

- Agency for Toxic Substances and Disease Registry www.atsdr.cdc.gov/
- Environmental Protection Agency www.epa.gov
- Centers for Disease Control and Prevention www.cdc.gov
- National Center for Environmental Health www.cdc.gov/nceh/
- National Institute of Environmental Health Sciences www.niehs.nih.gov/
- National Report on Human Exposure to Environmental Chemicals www.cdc.gov/exposurereport/

Non-government Sources of Information on Environmental Health

- American Academy of Environmental Medicine www.aaemonline.org/
- Collaborative on Health and the Environment www.healthandenvironment.org
- David Suzuki Foundation (health report series) www.davidsuzuki.org/health
- EcoHealth (journal) www.ecohealth.net/
- Environmental Health News www.EnvironmentalHealthNews.org
- Environmental Health Perspectives (free peer-reviewed journal) www.ehponline.org
- Greater Boston Physicians for Social Responsibility and the Science and Environmental Health Network www.agehealthy.org
- Harvard Medical School Center for Health and the Global Environment http://chge.med.harvard.edu/index.html
- PubMed (free database of medical journals) www.ncbi.nlm.nih.gov/pubmed/
- Science and Environmental Health Network www.sehn.org
- World Health Organization www.who.int/topics/environmental_health/en/

Print Sources of Information on Environmental Health

- Ackerman, F. 2008. *Poisoned for Pennies: The Economics of Toxics and Precaution.* Washington, DC: Island Press.

- Bullard, R.D., ed. 2005. *The Quest for Environmental Justice: Human Rights and the Politics of Pollution.* San Francisco: Sierra Club Books.

- Chivian, E., and A. Bernstein, eds. 2008. *Sustaining Life: How Human Health Depends on Biodiversity.* Oxford: Oxford University Press.

- Gavigan, C. 2008. *Healthy Child, Healthy World: Creating a Leaner, Greener, Safer Home.* New York: Penguin.

- Guidotti, T.L., and P. Gosselin, eds. 1999. *The Canadian Guide to Health and the Environment.* Edmonton: University of Alberta Press.

- Landrigan, P.J., H.L. Needleman, and M. Landrigan. 2001. *Raising Healthy Children in a Toxic World: 101 Smart Solutions for Every Family.* Emmaus, PA: Rodale.

- Prüss-Üstün, A., and C. Corvalán. 2006. *Preventing Disease Through Healthy Environments: Towards an Estimate of the Environmental Burden of Disease.* Geneva: World Health Organization.

- Soskolne, C.L., et al., eds. 2008. *Sustaining Life: Environmental and Human Health through Global Governance.* Lanham, MD: Lexington Books.

- Suzuki, D., and A. McConnell. 1997. *The Sacred Balance: Rediscovering Our Place in Nature.* Vancouver: Greystone.

2 The Outdoor Air We Breathe

Government Sources of Information on Outdoor Air

- Australian Department of the Environment, Water, Heritage and the Arts www.environment.gov.au/atmosphere/airquality/index.html

- Health Canada www.hc-sc.gc.ca/ewh-semt/air/out-ext/index-eng.php

- U.S. Environmental Protection Agency www.epa.gov/air/

Print Sources of Information on Outdoor Air

- American Lung Association. 2009. *State of the Air: 2009*. Washington, DC: ALA.

- Boyd, D.R. 2006. *The Air We Breathe: An International Comparison of Air Quality Standards and Guidelines*. Vancouver: David Suzuki Foundation.

- Canadian Medical Association. 2008. *No Breathing Room: National Illness Costs of Air Pollution*. Ottawa: CMA.

- Davis, D. 2002. *When Smoke Ran Like Water: Tales of Environmental Deception and the Battle Against Pollution*. New York: Basic Books.

- Doyle, J. 2000. *Taken for a Ride: Detroit's Big Three and the Politics of Pollution*. New York: Four Walls Eight Windows.

- Goodell, J. 2007. *Big Coal: The Dirty Secret Behind America's Energy Future*. Boston: Mariner Books.

- Tamminen, T. 2006. *Lives per Gallon: The True Cost of Our Oil Addiction*. Washington, DC: Island Press.

3 The Indoor Air We Breathe

Government Sources of Information on Indoor Air

- Australian Department of the Environment, Water, Heritage and the Arts www.environment.gov.au/atmosphere/airquality/indoorair/index.html

- Health Canada www.hc-sc.gc.ca/ewh-semt/air/in/index-eng.php

- U.S. Environmental Protection Agency www.epa.gov/iaq/index.html

Non-government Sources of Information on Indoor Air

- American Lung Association www.healthhouse.org

- Healthy House Institute www.HealthyHouseInstitute.com

4 The Food We Eat

Government Sources of Information on Fish
- Environment Canada www.ec.gc.ca/MERCURY/EN/fc.cfm
- Health Canada www.hc-sc.gc.ca/fn-an/securit/chem-chim/environ/ mercur/merc_fish_qa-poisson_qr-eng.php
- Food Standards Australia/New Zealand www.foodstandards.gov.au/_ srcfiles/brochure_mercury_in_fish_0304v2.pdf
- U.S. Environmental Protection Agency www.epa.gov/waterscience/fish/
- U.S. Environmental Protection Agency www.epa.gov/waterscience/fish/files/fisheng.pdf

Non-government Sources of Information on Food
- American Organic Consumers Association www.organicconsumers. org/btc/BuyingGuide.cfm
- Australian Farmers' Markets Association www.farmersmarkets.org.au
- Canadian Organic Growers www.cog.ca/buyorganic.html
- Eat Well Guide www.eatwellguide.org
- Farmers' Markets Canada www.farmersmarketscanada.ca
- Grass-fed meat and dairy products www.eatwild.com
- Organic Consumers Association www.organicconsumers.org
- Organic Food Directory for Australia www.organicfooddirectory.com.au
- U.S. farmers' markets www.localharvest.org

Print Sources of Information on Food
- Boyd, D.R. 2006. *The Food We Eat: An International Comparison of Pesticide Regulations.* Vancouver: David Suzuki Foundation.
- Hightower, J.M. 2009. *Diagnosis Mercury: Money, Politics and Poison.* Washington, DC: Island Press.

- Nestle, M. 2006. *What to Eat.* New York: North Point Press.

- Pollan, M. 2008. *In Defense of Food: An Eater's Manifesto.* New York: Penguin.

- Pollan, M. 2006. *The Omnivore's Dilemma: A Natural History of Four Meals.* New York: Penguin.

- Weil, A. 2000. *Eating Well for Optimum Health: The Essential Guide to Food, Diet, and Nutrition.* New York: Knopf.

- Willcox, B.J., D.C. Willcox, and M. Suzuki. 2000. *The Okinawa Program: How the World's Longest Lived People Achieve Everlasting Health, and How You Can Too.* New York: Three Rivers Press.

5 The Water We Drink

Government Sources of Information on Drinking Water
- Australia Department of Environment, Water, Heritage and the Arts www.environment.gov.au/water/index.html

- Australia's National Water Commission www.nwc.gov.au

- Health Canada www.hc-sc.gc.ca/ewh-semt/water-eau/drink-potab/index-eng.php

- U.S. Environmental Protection Agency www.epa.gov/safewater

    EPA. 2005. Bottled Water Basics

    EPA. 1999. Drinking Water and Health: What You Need to Know

    EPA. 2005. Filtration Facts

    EPA. 2003. Water on Tap: What You Need To Know

Print Sources of Information on Drinking Water
- Boyd, D.R. 2006. *The Water We Drink: An International Comparison of Drinking Water Standards.* Vancouver: David Suzuki Foundation.

- Hrudey, S.E., and E.J. Hrudey. 2004. *Safe Drinking Water: Lessons from Recent Outbreaks in Affluent Nations.* London: IWA Publishing.

- Royte, E. 2008. *Bottlemania: How Water Went on Sale and Why We Bought It.* New York: Bloomsbury.

6 The Things We Buy and Use

Non-government Sources of Information on Avoiding Hazardous Products
- Better Basics for the Home: Solutions for Less Toxic Living www.betterbasics.com
- Certified green cleaning products www.newdream.org/cleanschools/safelist.php
- Cosmetic Safety Database www.cosmeticsdatabase.com
- Environmental Home Center and Environmental Building Supplies www.ecohaus.com
- Green Depot www.GreenDepot.com
- Green Seal independent certification www.greenseal.org
- GreenSpec Directory, 7th ed. www.buildinggreen.com
- National Center for Healthy Housing www.nchh.org
- Healthy Home Institute www.healthyhomeinstitute.com
- Healthy Home Store www.thehealthiesthome.com

Print Sources of Information on Avoiding Hazardous Products
- Armstrong, L., G. Dauncey, and A. Wordsworth. 2007. *Cancer: 101 Solutions to a Preventable Epidemic.* Gabriola, BC: New Society.
- Baker, N. 2008. *The Body Toxic: How the Hazardous Chemistry of Everyday Things Threatens Our Health and Well-being.* New York: North Point Press.
- Blanc, P.D. 2007. *How Everyday Products Make People Sick: Toxins at Home and in the Workplace.* Berkeley: University of California Press.
- Center for Health, Environment, and Justice. 2008. *Pass Up the Poison Plastic: The PVC-Free Guide for Your Family and Home.*

- Dodd, D.L. 2005. *Home Safe Home: Protecting Yourself and Your Family From Everyday Toxics and Harmful Household Products*. New York: Tarcher.

- Ginsberg, G., and B. Toal. 2006. *What's Toxic, What's Not*. New York: Berkley Trade.

- Griffin, S. 2007. *CancerSmart Guide for Consumers*. Vancouver: Toxic Free Canada.

- Hollender, J., G. David, M. Hollender, and R. Doyle. 2006. *Naturally Clean: The Seventh Generation Guide to Safe & Healthy Non-toxic Cleaning*. Gabriola, BC: New Society.

- Institute for Agriculture and Trade Policy. 2008. *Smart Plastics Guide: Healthier Food Uses of Plastics*. Minneapolis, MN: IATP.

- Malkan, S. 2007. *Not Just a Pretty Face: The Ugly Side of the Beauty Industry*. Gabriola, BC: New Society Publishers.

- Smith, R., B. Lourie, and S. Dopp. 2009. *Slow Death by Rubber Duck: How the Toxic Chemistry of Everyday Life Affects Our Health*. Toronto: Knopf Canada.

7 The Physical Hazards We Face

Government Sources of Information on UV Radiation
- Australia Cancer Council www.cancer.org.au/cancersmartlifestyle/SunSmart.htm

- Australia National UV Index www.bom.gov.au/weather/national/charts/UV.shtml

- Environment Canada www.msc-smc.ec.gc.ca/education/uvindex/forecasts/forecastmap_e.html

- Health Canada www.hc-sc.gc.ca/ewh-semt/radiation/ultraviolet/index-eng.php

- U.S. Environmental Protection Agency UV Index www.epa.gov/sunwise/uvindex.html

8 Advocate for a Healthy Environment

- Carson, R. 1962. *Silent Spring*. Boston: Houghton Mifflin.

- Colborn, T., D. Dumanoski, and J.P. Myers. 1997. *Our Stolen Future: Are We Threatening Our Intelligence, Fertility, and Survival—A Scientific Detective Story*. New York: Penguin.

- Davis, D. 2007. *The Secret History of the War on Cancer*. New York: Basic Books.

- Markowitz, G., and D. Rosner. 2002. *Deceit and Denial: The Deadly Politics of Industrial Pollution*. Berkeley: University of California Press.

- Michaels, D. 2008. *Doubt Is Their Product: How Industry's Assault on Science Threatens Your Health*. Oxford: Oxford University Press.

- Schapiro, M. 2009. *Exposed: The Toxic Chemistry of Everyday Products and What's at Stake for American Power*. White River Junction, VT: Chelsea Green.

- Steingraber, S. 1998. *Living Downstream: A Scientist's Personal Investigation of Cancer and the Environment*. New York: Vintage.

9 Healthy Planet, Healthy People

- Daily, G.C., ed. 1997. *Nature's Services: Societal Dependence on Natural Ecosystems*. Washington, DC: Island Press.

- Frumkin, H., L. Frank, and R.J. Jackson. 2004. *Urban Sprawl and Public Health: Designing, Planning, and Building Healthy Communities*. Washington, DC: Island Press.

- Intergovernmental Panel on Climate Change. 2007. *Climate Change 2007: Synthesis Report*. Cambridge: Cambridge University Press.

- Layard, R. 2005. *Happiness: Lessons from a New Science*. London: Allen Lane.

- Louv, R. 2005. *Last Child in the Woods: Saving Our Children from Nature-deficit Disorder*. Chapel Hill, NC: Algonquin.

- Millennium Ecosystem Assessment. 2005. *Ecosystems and Human Well-being: Synthesis.* Washington, DC: Island Press.

- Nettle, D. 2005. *Happiness: The Science Behind Your Smile.* Oxford: Oxford University Press.

- Suzuki, D., and D. Boyd. 2008. *David Suzuki's Green Guide.* Vancouver: Greystone.

- Wilson, E.O. 2002. *The Future of Life.* New York: Knopf.

INDEX

Aamjiwnaang First Nation, 3, 39
acute toxicity, 85, 122–23, 126–27
aerosols and sprays, 53, 58, 60, 126, 127
agriculture. *See* farms and gardens
air cleaners and ventilation, 56, 58, 62,
    64, 65, 68–69
air filters, 64, 68, 71, 140
air fresheners, 21, 53, 57, 59, 136, 137
air pollution (indoor), 51–71; air cleaners,
    68–69; biological contaminants, 63–65;
    combustion products, 60, 62–63;
    prevention summary, 71; protecting
    children, 69–70; sources and health
    impacts, 51–65, 154; volatile organic
    compounds, 57–60. *See also* asbestos;
    radon; tobacco smoking
air pollution (outdoor), 29–49; industry
    denial, 15, 175; prevention and
    amelioration, 40–49; risk factors, 37–38,
    40; sources and health impacts, 29–35,
    37, 154; urban design and, 36
air quality indexes and reports, 40–43, 47
aldicarb, 85
allergies, 24, 52, 63–64, 90, 93, 125, 158
Alzheimer's disease, 122, 132, 154, 187
American Cancer Society, 54, 55, 171
American Lung Association, 55, 171
animal dander and wastes, 63
antibacterial products, 121, 129
antibiotics, 74, 76, 78–79, 89, 131, 177, 186
arsenic, 144; developmental neurotoxin, 61;
    in drinking water, 100, 101, 109, 110, 115;
    in foods, 74, 79, 81; in pressure-treated
    lumber, 46, 122, 124; standards for, 106,
    177; in tobacco smoke, 53; in toys, 120
artificial sweeteners, 90
asbestos, 12–13, 65–67, 120, 144, 175, 177
asthma: and air pollution (indoor), 52–53,

54, 60, 62, 63, 69, 71; and air pollution
    (outdoor), 31, 32, 33, 35, 38, 43, 44, 47;
    and consumer products, 127, 136
Atlanta Olympics, air quality, 31
atrazine, 11–12, 87
Australia, policies: air quality index and
    standards, 42, 43; on asbestos, 177;
    asthma prevalence and costs, 52;
    climate change impacts, 185; on
    consumer products, 177; on developing
    nations, 179; environmental NGOs,
    172; environmental rights, 174;
    environmental standards, 195; and
    ethnicity, 23; and Europe, compared, 164,
    177; on flame retardants, 26, 177; on food
    coloring, 93; illness from contaminated
    water, 100; on labeling, 90; on lead, 134;
    mortality from environmental hazards,
    12; on nuclear waste, 164–65; on PBDES,
    139–40; on pesticides, 86–87, 177;
    on phthalates, 177; on radon, 55;
    skin cancer risks, 153
Australian Lung Foundation, 55, 172

backyard burning, 46, 77, 145
benzene: as air pollutant, 30, 31, 34;
    avoidance strategies, 58; carcinogen, 11,
    19, 30, 144; defended by industry, 175;
    standards for, 11, 19; in tobacco smoke, 53
Bernstein, Aaron, 9, 173, 183
beryllium, 144, 175
biodiversity, and human health, 184,
    186–89, 193–94, 196
biological hazards, 19, 21, 63–65.
    See also microbiological hazards
bird flu, 76, 190
birth defects, 35, 39, 120, 123, 135,
    136, 138, 139

hantavirus, 64
Health Canada, 134
hearing loss, 159–60
heart disease, 32, 35, 37, 53–54, 76, 132–33.
    See also cardiovascular diseases
heavy metals, 31, 61, 76, 104, 107–9,
    132, 135, 178. *See also specific metals*
Helena, Montana, 70–71
hepatitis A, 87, 100
hexachlorobenzene, 11, 135
hexavalent chromium, 120, 165, 175
Hinkley, California, 165
Hong Kong, air quality, 31
hormone disruptors.
    See endocrine disruptors
hormones, 14, 18, 74, 76, 79, 86, 160, 177
house dust and mites, 63, 64, 67, 70, 138,
    139–41. *See also* particulate pollution
houseplants, as air cleaners, 68–69
human immunodeficiency virus (HIV), 190
human physiology, 9–10, 29–30,
    73–74, 97–98
human rights, environmental, 25,
    174, 176, 178–79
humidity control, 64, 71
hyperactivity disorder, 16, 93, 94
hypospadias, 39, 120

immune system disorders: from consumer
    products, 26, 135, 138, 140; from foods,
    77, 82, 83, 88; from noise, 160; as risk
    factor, 23, 78, 100, 101, 111, 112; from
    UV radiation, 152–53; and vitamin D, 157
indoor sports facilities, 71
industrial facilities, 30, 44, 98
infectious diseases. *See* microbiological
    hazards; *specific diseases and pathogens*;
    zoonoses
International Union Against Cancer, 54

kidney disorders, 57, 78, 100, 115, 132, 140

lead: abatement of, 133; blood levels, 18–19,
    61, 134; in bottled water, 110; and brain

dysfunction, 154; children's exposure,
    13, 24, 61, 120; in consumer products
    and toys, 120, 121, 132–34; defended by
    industry, 175; in developing nations, 180;
    in gasoline, 15; standards and testing, 116,
    142, 178; in water supplies, 107, 113–14
life expectancy, 28, 75
Listeria, 74, 78, 87
liver disorders, 57, 100, 140
London, smog disaster, 31
Love Canal, New York, 164
lung diseases. *See* respiratory illnesses

malathion, 16
May, Elizabeth, 164
meat and dairy products, 76–81
medications, 109, 115, 121, 131, 186–88
mental health, 61, 160, 184, 193–94, 196
mercury: in consumer products, 121,
    134–35; defended by industry, 175;
    in developing nations, 180;
    developmental impacts, 28, 34,
    61; in fish, 73–74, 82, 83, 84;
    methyl mercury, 82; sex ratio
    impacts, 39; in toys, 120
Merlini, David, 29
methylation, 27
methyl bromide, 158
methylene chloride, 58
microbiological hazards, 63–65, 78,
    99–101, 107, 109, 110, 111, 129
Millennium Ecosystem Assessment, 188
Milwaukee, Wisconsin, 99
molds and mildew, 52, 63–65, 71
monosodium glutamate (MSG), 90
Montreal Protocol, 180–81
mortality, 12, 32, 33, 35, 75, 99–100
mothballs, 58, 59, 123
motor vehicles: accidents, 149–51; air
    quality inside, 44–45; exhaust pollutants,
    30–31, 60, 71; fuel efficiency, 174;
    idling, 47, 60, 62; industry tactics, 15,
    174, 175; protecting children, 161

nanotechnology products, 121, 130–31
National Collaborating Centre for
    Environmental Health, 134
National Institute for Occupational
    Safety and Health, 58
National Safety Council, 56, 150
National Sanitation Foundation, 108
neurological disorders, 12, 13, 154; from
    air pollution, 35, 57, 61; from consumer
    products, 122, 123; from food, 86;
    from water pollution, 101.
    See also specific disorders
Nipah virus, 190
nitrates, 109, 114
nitrogen oxides, 30, 31, 33–34,
    43, 44–45, 60, 62
noise, 159–61, 162
North American Free Trade
    Agreement (NAFTA), 178
Norway, 26, 176, 195

obesity, 14, 74–76, 187
Okinawa, Japan, 154
Olestra, 90
omega-3 fatty acids, 81, 84
organic foods and practices, 16,
    91, 94, 124, 126
organophosphates, 16
Our Stolen Future, 165, 173
outdoor activities, 38, 40–48, 194, 196
ozone, 15, 31–32, 33, 152, 156, 158, 180–81

paints, 34, 57, 58, 67, 69–70,
    133–34, 142, 143
parabens, 124–25
Parkinson's disease, 86, 122, 132, 154, 187
particulate pollution, 30–32, 60,
    62, 64, 68, 71, 140
perchlorate, 11
perchloroethylene, 58, 59, 127
perfluorinated chemicals (PFCs),
    11, 18, 121, 140–41
persistent organic pollutants (POPs),
    14, 15, 76, 77, 95, 180. *See also* dioxins

pesticides: aldicarb, 85; atrazine, 11–12, 87;
    borax, 123; childhood exposure, 18,
    94; chlorpyrifos, 16; comparison of
    standards, 177; as consumer products,
    121, 122–24; cosmetic use of, 178;
    2,4-D, 178; defended by industry, 15,
    175; dibromochloropropane, 174;
    in foods, 85–87, 88, 91, 94; health
    impacts, 85, 154; hexachlorobenzene,
    11, 135; malathion, 16; methyl
    bromide, 158; mothballs, 58, 59, 123;
    organophosphates, 16; regulation of,
    178; sex ratio impacts, 39; vinclozolin,
    27; in water, 101, 107
phenylenediamine, 125
phthalates: in bottled water, 110; in
    consumer products, 59, 121, 124–25,
    135, 136–37, 138; defended by industry,
    175; standards for, 142, 177
physical hazards, 149–62; cell phones,
    158–59; defined, 19–20; motor vehicles,
    149–51; noise, 159–61; power lines,
    158–59, 162; prevention summary,
    161–62; radiation, 151–59; ultraviolet
    radiation, 109, 152–58, 162; X-rays,
    145, 152, 158–59
Plain, Ron, 3
plastics, 110, 137–39, 143, 146. *See also*
    bisphenol A (BPA); dioxins; phthalates;
    polycarbonate; polyvinyl chloride (PVC)
poisoning. *See* acute toxicity
pollen, 32, 63, 68
polybrominated diphenyl ethers (PBDEs).
    See flame retardants
polycarbonate, 137, 138
polychlorinated biphenyls (PCBs):
    prohibition of, 120; sex ratio impacts, 39;
    sources and health impacts, 61, 82–83,
    84, 135; and triclosan, 129; ubiquity of,
    15, 23, 35; water treatment for, 107
polycyclic aromatic hydrocarbons (PAHs),
    31, 34–35, 62, 107, 144
polyvinyl chloride (PVC), 59, 121, 135–36
population growth, 184

2,3,7,8-TCDD, 77
Thornton, Joe, 135
3M Company, 141
tobacco smoking, 53–55, 58, 69, 70–71, 175
toluene, 58, 61, 109, 124–25, 126
Toxic Substances Control Act, 120
toxic waste, 21, 59, 164
Toxoplasma, 78, 100
trade agreements, 178, 179–80
transportation, 30, 43–45, 47, 150–51, 178, 191. *See also* motor vehicles
tributyltin (TBT), 14
trichloroethylene, 99, 127
triclosan, 129–30, 148

ultraviolet light, 109, 152–58, 162
United Nations Millennium Development Goals, 179
United States, policies: air pollution costs, 48; air quality index and standards, 42, 43; on asbestos, 177; asthma prevalence and costs, 52; bottled water consumption, 99; cataract risks, 153; on consumer products, 120, 125, 177; on developing nations, 179; environmental NGOs, 171–72; environmental rights, 174; environmental standards, 195; and ethnicity, 23; and Europe, compared, 164, 177; on flame retardants, 26, 177; on food coloring, 92–93; illness from contaminated water, 99–100; on labeling, 90; on lead, 142; mortality from environmental hazards, 12; on PBDES, 139–40; on pesticides, 86–87, 177; on phthalates, 137, 142, 177; public water supplies, 103; on radon, 55; skin cancer risks, 153; traffic accidents, 150
urban design, 36
U.S. Consumer Product Safety Commission, 134
U.S. Environmental Protection Agency, 56, 63, 71, 105, 120, 141
U.S. Institute of Medicine, 163

vehicle exhaust. *See under* motor vehicles
vinclozolin, 27
vinyl chloride, 53, 135, 144, 175. *See also* polyvinyl chloride (PVC)
vitamins, 88, 152, 157
volatile organic compounds (VOCS), 33, 34, 45, 57–60, 109

Walkerton, Ontario, 99
waterborne pathogens, 99–101
water pollution, 97–117; arsenic, 100, 101, 109, 110, 115; boil water advisories, 112; bottled water, 98–99, 109–10; chemical contaminants, 100, 101–2, 109, 114, 144; fresh water supply, 98; lead, 100, 107, 113–14; microbiological contaminants, 99–101, 107, 109, 110, 111, 129; prevention and amelioration, 102–9, 115–17; public vs. private supplies, 99–100, 102–10; radiological contaminants, 100, 102, 110; sources and health impacts, 20–21, 98, 99–102; treatment (home), 107–10, 111, 113, 115; water quality tests, 103–4, 106; wells, 101, 102–10, 114, 115
West Nile virus, 185, 189
wildfires, 46–47
wildlife, 26, 98, 101, 129, 131, 139, 187
Wilson, E.O., 186
Wingfield, Eileen Wani, 164–65
Woburn, Massachusetts, 99
wood products, 46, 58, 120, 122, 124
wood smoke, 31, 46, 60, 62
workers' health and safety, 65, 86, 92, 144–45, 174, 176
World Cancer Research Fund, 76
World Health Organization (WHO), 12, 65, 66, 75, 77, 163, 185

X-rays, 145, 152, 158–59
xylene, 34, 109

zoonoses, 185, 188–89, 190. *See also* *specific diseases and pathogens*

The David Suzuki Foundation

The David Suzuki Foundation works through science and education to protect the diversity of nature and our quality of life, now and for the future.

With a goal of achieving sustainability within a generation, the Foundation collaborates with scientists, business and industry, academia, government, and nongovernmental organizations. We seek the best research to provide innovative solutions that will help build a clean, competitive economy that does not threaten the natural services that support all life.

The Foundation is a federally registered independent charity that is supported with the help of over 50,000 individual donors across Canada and around the world.

We invite you to become a member. For more information on how you can support our work, please contact us:

The David Suzuki Foundation
219–2211 West 4th Avenue
Vancouver, BC
Canada V6K 4S2
www.davidsuzuki.org
contact@davidsuzuki.org
Tel: 604-732-4228
Fax: 604-732-0752

Checks can be made payable to The David Suzuki Foundation.
All donations are tax-deductible.

Canadian charitable registration: (BN) 12775 6716 RR0001

U.S. charitable registration: #94-3204049

Other titles from the David Suzuki Foundation and Greystone Books

- *Lakeland: Journeys into the Soul of Canada* by Allan Casey
- *The Big Picture: Reflections on Science, Humanity, and a Quickly Changing Planet* by David Suzuki and Dave Robert Taylor
- *A Good Catch: Sustainable Seafood Recipes From Canada's Top Chefs* by Jill Lambert
- *Tar Sands: Dirty Oil and the Future of a Continent* by Andrew Nikiforuk
- *David Suzuki's Green Guide* by David Suzuki and David R. Boyd
- *Bees: Nature's Little Wonders* by Candace Savage
- *The Hot Topic: What We Can Do about Global Warming* by Gabrielle Walker and Sir David King
- *A Passion for This Earth: Writers, Scientists, and Activists Explore Our Relationship with Nature and the Environment* edited by Michelle Benjamin
- *The Great Lakes: The Natural History of a Changing Region* by Wayne Grady
- *The Sacred Balance: Rediscovering Our Place in Nature* by David Suzuki, Amanda McConnell, and Adrienne Mason
- *An Enchantment of Birds: Memories from a Birder's Life* by Richard Cannings
- *Wisdom of the Elders: Native and Scientific Ways of Knowing about Nature* by Peter Knudtson and David Suzuki
- *Rockies: A Natural History* by Richard Cannings
- *Wild Prairie: A Photographer's Personal Journey* by James R. Page
- *Prairie: A Natural History* by Candace Savage
- *Tree: A Life Story* by David Suzuki and Wayne Grady
- *The Sacred Balance: A Visual Celebration of Our Place in Nature* by David Suzuki and Amanda McConnell with Maria DeCambra
- *From Naked Ape to Superspecies: Humanity and the Global Eco-Crisis* by David Suzuki and Holly Dressel
- *The David Suzuki Reader* by David Suzuki
- *Good News for a Change: How Everyday People Are Helping the Planet* by David Suzuki and Holly Dressel